A Guide to
Ethnic Health Collections
in the United States

Recent Titles in
Bibliographies and Indexes in Medical Studies

Federal Information Sources in Health and Medicine: A Selected
Annotated Bibliography
Mary Glen Chitty, compiler, with the assistance of Natalie Schatz

Viruses and Reproduction: A Bibliography
Ernest L. Abel, compiler

The History of Cancer: An Annotated Bibliography
James S. Olson, compiler

New Literature On Fetal Alcohol Exposure and Effects: A Bibliography,
1983–1988
Ernest L. Abel, compiler

Sociodemographic Factors in the Epidemiology of Multiple Sclerosis:
An Annotated Bibliography
George W. Lowis, compiler

Prostitutes in Medical Literature: An Annotated Bibliography
Sachi Sri Kantha, compiler

Vital and Health Statistics Series: An Annotated Checklist and Index
to the Publications of the "Rainbow Series"
Jim Walsh and A. James Bothmer, compilers

Medicine in Great Britain from the Restoration to the Nineteenth Century,
1660–1800: An Annotated Bibliography
Samuel J. Rogal, compiler

Treatment of Cocaine Abuse: An Annotated Bibliography
John J. Miletich, compiler

AIDS: A Multimedia Sourcebook
John J. Miletich, compiler

Depression: A Multimedia Sourcebook
John J. Miletich, compiler

Injury Prevention for Young Children: A Research Guide
Bonnie L. Walker, compiler

A Guide to
Ethnic Health Collections
in the United States

Compiled by
TYSON GIBBS

Bibliographies and Indexes in Medical Studies,
Number 13

GREENWOOD PRESS
Westport, Connecticut • London

Library of Congress Cataloging-in-Publication Data

Gibbs, Tyson.
    A guide to ethnic health collections in the United States /
compiled by Tyson Gibbs.
        p.   cm.—(Bibliographies and indexes in medical studies,
    ISSN 0896–6591 ; no. 13)
    Rev. ed. of: Ethnic health collections in the United States. East
Point, Ga. : Jamilla Powers, 1993.
    Includes bibliographical references and index.
    ISBN 0–313–29740–1 (alk. paper)
    1. Minorities—Health and hygiene—United States—Library
resources—Directories. 2. Minorities—Health and hygiene—United
States—Archival resources—Directories. I. Gibbs, Tyson. Ethnic
health collections in the United States. II. Title. III. Series.
    [DNLM 1. Ethnic Groups—history—United States—directories.
2. Information Centers—United States—directories. 3. Public
Health—history—United States—directories. Z 675 .M4G444g 1996]
Z6675. M68G52   1996
[RA448.4]
016.3621'0425'0973—dc20
DNLM/DLC   95–50402

British Library Cataloguing in Publication Data is available.

Library of Congress Catalog Card Number: 95–50402
ISBN: 0–313–29740–1
ISSN: 0896–6591

First published in 1996

Greenwood Press, 88 Post Road West, Westport, CT 06881
An imprint of Greenwood Publishing Group, Inc.

Printed in the United States of America

The paper used in this book complies with the
Permanent Paper Standard issued by the National
Information Standards Organization (Z39.48–1984).

10 9 8 7 6 5 4 3 2 1

Contents

Introduction

The United States of America is a mosaic of different ethnic groups whose cultural background provides a benchmark for the types of health issues that might affect individuals within that group. For these minorities it is often difficult to gain a complete understanding of group health problems because the types of studies needed, the kinds of research tools and the lack of a methodology for systematically monitoring medical problems are unavailable.

What evidence is available for understanding disease and illness within these groups paints a bleak picture if contrasted within the dominant Caucasian culture population.

The important ethnic minorities are generally identified as those persons of African American, Hispanic, Pacific Asian American, Native American, Native Hawaiian, Alaska Native or Samoan descent. It must be clearly understood that not all minorities suffer from the same health problems nor do these groups have the same or even similar mortality rates.

What makes these different ethnic groups interesting is that much of their health status is intricately bound to differences in lifestyle behavior. These lifestyle differences can be attributed to cultural behavior found within each group.

Health-seeking activities, health promotion behavior, doctors visits, medication taking behavior and use of alternate medicines can all be linked to the ethnic templates that make each individual part of the larger whole.

Similarly, each group is composed of many other identifiable, smaller ethnic groups that make the examination of health issues problematic. For example, Native Americans are represented by over 300 different peoples. For the sake of convenience, the entire population is called "Native Americans."

Each of these peoples-- Cheyenne, Hopi, Cherokee, Navaho, Shoshone, etc. -- have different ways in which they resolve health issues affecting their group.

Hispanics are made up of Cubans, Puerto Ricans, or Mexican Americans. Each of these groups has developed ways of resolving health problems that may or may not have similar characteristics.

Clearly ethnic heritage plays a key role in the development of and resolution of health problems.

DEFINITIONS

People classified as Caucasians are represented by groups as diverse as peoples from France, Germany, Ireland, Spain, Italy, Turkey, Russia, Poland, Portugal, Romania or Scotland. There are approximately 199,686,070 people who are classified as Caucasians in the United States and account for 74% of the United States total population.

Individuals called African-Americans or Black people encompass such groups as Native Born Americans whose ancestors were African slaves, persons from the Caribbean Basin or West Indies, all types of peoples from Sub-Sahara Africa, and dark pigmented individuals from Brazil or Cuba. Although as diverse as other broadly classified ethnic groups, these individuals are lumped into this one category. They number about 29,986,060 persons or 12.9% of the total population.

Native Americans or American Indians are considered the original aboriginal Indian or Eskimo peoples of North and South America. Remaining in the United States are only 1,959,234 or less than 1% of the total population. This small number covers about 355 different tribal groups.

Pacific Asian Americans or people of Asian American descent, are usually defined as persons from: China, Japan, Vietnam, Filipinos, Cambodia, or Thailand and other southeast and Pacific region countries. 7,293,662 Asian people in the United States account for 2.9% of the total population.

Hispanics are people whose native tongue is the Spanish language. Representative of the persons in this group are Mexicans, Cubans, Puerto Ricans, Panamanians, and Spanish-speaking peoples from South America. There are 22,359,059 people in this category or 9.0% of the total United States population.

GEOGRAPHIC LOCATION

Data from the 1991 Census of Population Statistics show that some of all of these ethnic groups live in every state within America. However, some racial groups outnumber others by extreme numbers in some states.

People classified as Caucasians (32.8%) and people of African-American descent (52.8%) are disproportionately located in the South. Native Americans (47.6%) and Asians (55.7%) are located in the North East. Hispanics (45.2%), to a large degree, are located in the West.

The top five states of residence for Caucasians are: California (10.3%), New York (6.7%), Texas (6.4%), Florida (5.4%), and Pennsylvania (5.3%).

The top five states of residence for African-Americans are: New York (9.5%), California (7.4%), Texas (6.7%), Florida (5.9%), and Georgia (5.8%).

The top five states of residence for Native Americans are: Oklahoma (12.9%), California (12.4%), Arizona (10.4%), New Mexico (6.9%), and Alaska (4.4%).

The top five states of residence for Pacific Asian Americans are: California (39.1%), New York (9.5%), Hawaii (9.4%), Texas (4.9%), and Illinois (3.9%).

The top five states for Hispanic Americans are: California (34.4%), Texas (19.4%), New York (9.9%), Florida (7.0%), and Illinois (4.0%).

CAUSE OF DEATH

Data from "Health, United States 1991" shows that the top five causes of death vary by ethnic group and gender within each ethnic group.

Males

For persons classified as Caucasians, the top causes of death for males are: disease of the heart (325,397), malignant neoplasm (228,301), accidents and adverse effects (52,691), cerebrovascular disease (48,563), and chronic obstructive pulmonary disease (44,046).

For African American males, the top five causes of death are: diseases of the heart (933,321), malignant meoplasm (31,452), accidents and adverse effects (9,503), homicide and legal intervention (8,888), and cerebrovascular disease (7,739).

The top five causes of death for Native American males are: diseases of the heart (1,184), accidents and adverse effects (885), malignant neoplasm (706), chronic liver disease and cirrhosis (214), and suicide (197).

The top five causes of death for Pacific Asian males are: diseases of the heart (3,240), malignant neoplasm (2,831), cerebrovascular disease (821), accidents and adverse effects (8070), and pneumonia and influenza (473).

Females

In contrast, the top five causes of death for Caucasian American females are diseases of the heart (323,469), malignant neoplasm (205,855), cerebrovascular disease (76,953), pneumonia and influenza (36,961), and chronic obstructive pulmonary disease (33,835).

The top five causes of death for African-American females are diseases of the heart (39,110), malignant neoplasm (24,112), cerebrovascular disease (10,240), diabetes mellitus (4,883), and accidents and adverse effects (3,901).

The top five causes of death for Native American females are diseases of the heart (860), malignant neoplasm (612), accidents and adverse effects (318), diabetes mellitus (211), and cerebrovascular disease (181).

The top five causes of death for Pacific Asian American females are malignant neoplasm (2,236), diseases of the heart (2,186), cerebrovascular disease (846), accidents and adverse effects (442), and pneumonia and influenza (328).

SUMMARY

One will note that many of the same diseases are found in the top five causes of death for the different ethnic groups. There are two key points to remember. First, while the diseases are the same, both the proportion and severity of the disease is different for each group. Second, many of the root causes of the disease may vary by group because of culture. Ethnic culture provides the template for making decisions about eating habits, weight control, exercise, doctor visits and decisions about when to seek medical attention. All these matters affect disease outcome.

THE REPOSITORIES

Ethnic collections relating to health have been identified at many repositories throughout the country. For the most part, however, much of the material remains uncataloged, and according to many librarians, there are no plans to seek new materials. With exceptions, such as Howard University, Moorland-Springarn Research Center and Health Science Library, Schomburg Collection in New York, Fisk University Library Special Collection and the University of Louisville Kornhauser Health Science Library, most of the material on health, medicine and ethnic groups is scattered throughout larger collections.

Although these collections are an invaluable source of material by and about minority groups, individually or collectively, they do not constitute a comprehensive collection on ethnic medical history. The major gaps in existing ethnic health history collections are: 1) many records are uncataloged and generally unavailable for public use; 2) the lack of consistent internal research and consistent development of these collections; and 3) many collections have limited scope, focusing on single individuals, city or state health activities, and limit materials to those acquired as gifts.

In the analysis of the materials describing ethnic health collections at repositories, it was discovered that over 50% of the collections were uncataloged and generally unavailable for public use. The ability to identify, retrieve, display, and publicize the materials in a collection are important hallmarks toward developing a significant and useful health collection. It is also equally important that there be a database for the collection so that solicited materials and those given without solicitation will have a place in the collection.

ETHNIC HEALTH COLLECTIONS

Searching for historical materials related to health and ethnic minority groups in the United States is a tedious and difficult task. While the major libraries have some of this information, there is also important information at the local level. To date, while the interest has grown in issues that explore questions of the health of ethnic minority groups in the past, little has been done to learn where these materials are. The purpose of this book is to identify the various collections, their content, and their location relative to African Americans, Hispanics, Native Americans, and Pacific Asian Americans. What we have found is that there is more material available on all groups than we anticipated. The major problem is that much of it is uncatalogued and aggregated with other collection materials. Thus, in many instances, the researcher can often provide a useful service for a library as he or she searches through uncatalogued collections locating particular materials.

Questionnaires were mailed to state libraries, state archives, public and private libraries, college and university libraries, selected hospitals, libraries of schools of medicine and public health, and government agencies annually. More than two-thirds of these questionnaires were returned. The results are the basis of this book and it represents one of the first volumes to collect such information. It would not be possible, however, without the enthusiastic cooperation of the libraries which responded to our questionnaire.

The main part of the book consists of the various collections, arranged first by state, then by ethnic group as the subheading, followed by name and location of the library, and an alphabetical listing of the collection. The Appendix include the questionnaire and a complete list of libraries contacted. A bibliography lists additional sources of information about ethnic health.

We strongly recommend a letter of inquiry or a phone call to the perspective library before a visit is attempted. Many collections are closed to the public, but open to researchers.

THE REPOSITORIES

ALABAMA

African Americans

State of Alabama
Department of Archives and History
P.O. Box 300100
624 Washington Avenue
Montgomery, Alabama 36130
(205)242-4152
> Status: permanent
> Update: none
> Dated: 1847-1939
> Volume: unreported

> Alabama Insane Hospitals Reports, 1901-1964, including reports from the Hospital for African American patients, Mt. Vernon/Searcy.

> Reports from Freedman's Hospital in Talladega, 1869-1974.

Tuskegee University Archives
Tuskegee Institute, Alabama 36088
> Status: Permanent
> Update: none
> Dated: 1912-1972
> Volume: 150 books; 15,000 other documents (journals, studies, manuscripts)
> Library Hours:
> 8:00 a.m.-10:00 p.m. Monday-Thursday
> 8:00 a.m.- 4:30 p.m. Friday
> 9:00 a.m.- 1:00 p.m. Saturday
> 2:00 p.m.- 6:00 p.m. Sunday

Archives Hours:
8:00 a.m.-4:30 p.m. Monday-Friday

Eugene H. Dibble Papers, 1923-1968. Practiced in general medicine and was a member of the John A. Andrew Clinical Society. Collection composed of manuscripts.

Louise Brisco Trigg, 1945-1960. Worked in area of social work. Collection composed of manuscripts and pamphlets.

National Negro Health News, 1943-1950. Volumes 11-18.

The Tuskegee Syphilis Study and Ad Hoc Advisory Panel, 1936-1972.

Negro Yearbook Clippings File, 1912-1966. Twenty-five cartons. Published at Tuskegee Institute.

History of the V.A. Medical Hospital Clipping File. Five cartons of clippings. Hospital site, at Tuskegee, Alabama.

Native Americans

University of Alabama at Birmingham
Lister Hill Library of the Health Sciences
Birmingham, Alabama 25294
        Status: permanent
        Update: annual
        Dated: 1886 - mid 1900's
        Volume: 15-20 documents

Reynolds Historical Library, Alabama Museum of the Health Sciences. The Reynolds Historical Library is a collection of rare and important works in the history of the health sciences. The Alabama Museum of the Health Sciences covers memorabilia related to the history of the health sciences in Alabama. These collections have a few books about medicine among the Native Americans.

ALASKA

Pacific Asian Americans

Department of Education
State Archives and Records Management Services
141 Willoughby Avenue
Juneau, Alaska 99801
(907)466-2270
>   Status: permanent annual as scheduled
>   Dated: 1960 - present-various, 1895
>   Volume: 52 cubic feet

RG 101 Territorial Governor Reports. Covers health services and conditions of Alaska natives. Included are letters and photographs.

RG 108/RG 6 Territorial States Department of Health. Covers delivery of health services to Alaska natives; included are letters, reports, articles and forms.

ARIZONA

General

Arizona State Archive
Department of Library, Archives and Public Records
3rd Floor, Capitol
Phoenix, Arizona 85007
>   Status: permanent
>   Update: monthly
>   Dated: 1860 - present
>   Volume: 104,000 documents

Arizona History. References to studies and statements concerning ethnic minorities dispersed throughout collection. Collection consists of letters, articles and newspapers.

ARKANSAS

No Collections Reported

CALIFORNIA

General

California State Archives
1020 "O" Street
Sacramento, California 95814
       Status: permanent
       Update: as needed
       Dated: 1898-1940
       Volume: 5 cubic feet
       Hours: 9:30 a.m. - 4:00 p.m.

California Departments of Public Health, Social Welfare and the Board of Professional and Vocational Standards. These collections are made up of agency-related data including references to immigrant health care, and a minority index of deceased physicians from the Board of Medical Examiners. The collection media is manuscripts.

San Francisco Psychoanalytic Institute Library
2420 Sutler Street
San Francisco, California 94115
       Status: permanent
       Update: monthly
       Dated: 1928 - present
       Volume: 4,000 titles, 90 journals, 10,000 reprints
       Hours: 9:00 a.m. - 5:00 p.m.

Pravdian Psychoanalysis, 1928 to present. Contains a few books on racism and cultural differences. Books and articles. Jews, Holocaust survivors, psychotherapy.

Pacific Asian Americans

University of California, San Francisco Library
San Francisco, California 94143
> Status: permanent
> Update: monthly
> Dated: unreported
> Volume: 10,000+ documents

Oriental Medicine Collection. This collection contains books, pamphlets and other materials related to the health sciences of the Orient, especially China, Korea, Japan and some Southeast indigenous to Asian countries. Its holdings include both historical and contemporary books and materials on the subject written in various dialects, native languages, as well as western languages.

COLORADO

General

State of Colorado
Division of Archives and Public Record
1313 Sherman Street, Room 1B-20
Denver, Colorado 80203
(303)866-2358
> Status: permanent
> Update: none
> Dated: 1964 - 1983
> Volume: 42 documents
> Hours: 9:00 - 4:45, Monday-Friday

Colorado department of health, division of migrant health publications concerning housing, sanitation and health care for migrant workers.

CONNECTICUT

No Collections Reported

DELAWARE

No Collection Reported

DISTRICT OF COLUMBIA

General

Association of American Medical Colleges - Archives
Suite 200, One Dupont Circle, N.W.
Washington, DC 20036
       Status: permanent
       Update: annual
       Dated: 1968-1985
       Volume: 27 documents

Records of Health Professions Education for Minority Students in the
US, 1968-1985. Describes opportunities for minorities in medicine
applications to and admissions in U.S. medical schools 1968-1985.

Georgetown University Medical Center
John Vinton Dahlgren Memorial Library
3900 Reservoir Road, N.W.
Washington, DC 20007
       Status: permanent
       Update: periodic
       Dated: 1932-present
       Volume: 50 documents
Collection volumes deal with the health of African Americans,
Hispanics, and Native Americans.

African Americans

The Library of Congress
Manuscript Division
Washington, DC 20540
  Status: permanent
  Update: annual
  Dated: unreported
  Volume: unreported

Louise Bates Ames-Frances. Collection consists of papers related to psychological development of African American and Caucasian American children.

Benjamin Barr Lindsey. Papers in this collection are concerned with sex education and birth control.
Margaret Sanger. Papers on African American working-class women and family planning.

NAACP and National Urban League. Papers on such health issues as infant mortality, sickle-cell anemia, and tuberculosis.

Booker T. Washington Papers. Materials relating to health and hygiene of African Americans in rural areas. Some files relating to National Negro Health Week.

Nannie Helen Burroughs Papers. Some materials relating to health and hygiene in the African American community.

Howard University
Health Sciences Library
P.O. Box 533 600 W Street, N.W.
Washington, DC 20059
  Status: permanent
  Update: monthly
  Dated: 1825 - present
  Volume: unreported
  Hours: 8:30 a.m.-12:00 midnight, Monday-Saturday
  I.D. required (drivers licenses, passport etc.)

The collection consists of vertical file folders containing photographs, reprints, newspaper clippings, and press releases about notable African Americans in the health sciences.

1.   Carolina V. Still Anderson, M.D., 1849-1919. One of the two pioneer African American women physicians. Materials include biographical sketch.

2.   William Harry Barns, M.D., 1887-1945.
        Otolaryngology. Materials include article.
        Montague W. Cobbs, M.D., Ph.D., 1904-date. Anatomy, Anthropology, Medical History, Materials include articles.

3.   Green Vardiman Black, 1836-1913. Dentist-Oral Surgeon. Materials include one article.

4.   Ulysses Grant Dailey, M.D., 1885-1961. Surgery. Materials include articles.

5.   Russell A. Dixon, Sr., D.D.S., 1898-1976. Dentistry. Materials include articles clippings, and photographs.

6.   Charles Richard Drew, 1904-1950. Surgery, Blood Bank Materials include bust, articles, clippings, and photographs.

7.   Clifton O. Dummett, 1919-date. Dentistry, Youngest Dean. Materials include article and clippings.

8.   Edgar N. Duncan, 1932-date. Assistant Surgeon General U.S. Public Health Service Pharmacists. Materials include articles.

9.   Ida Gray, D.D.S., 1867-? First Negro Woman Dentist. Materials include clippings

10.   Margaret E. Grigsby, M.D., 1930-date. Topical Medicine. Materials include articles.

11.   William A. Hinton, 1883-1959. Serology, Bacteriology. Materials include articles.

12. Theodore K. Lawless, 1892-1971. Dermatology. Materials include articles.

13. LeSalle D. Leffall, Jr., 1930-date. Surgery, Cancer. Materials include articles.

14. Miles Vandahurst Lynk, M.D., 1871-date. Founder of First Negro Medical Journal. Material includes articles.

15. Mary Eliza Mahoney, 1845-1926. First Negro Nurse. Materials include clippings.

16. Hildrus A. Poindexter, M.D., M.P.H., Ph.D., 1901-date. Preventive Medicine Community Health. Materials include books and articles.

17. Alvin F. Poussaint, M.D., 1934-date. Psychiatry. Materials include article, and clippings.

18. John Sweat Rock, M.D., Esq., 1825-1866. Surgery, Law, Dentistry. Material includes articles.

19. Roland B. Scott, M.D., 1909-date. Pediatrics, Sickle Cell Anemia. Materials include articles, and clippings.

20. Jeanne C. Sinkford, D.D.S., 1933-date. Dentist; First African American Woman Dean. Materials include photograph, and clippings.

21. Daniel Hale Williams, M.D., 1858-1931. Surgeon. Materials include book, bust, clippings, and reprints.

22. Louis Thompkins Wright, M.D., 1891-1952. Surgeon.

Howard University
Moorland-Springarn Research Center
Manuscript Department
Washington, DC 20059
 Status: permanent
 Update: monthly
 Dated: 1852-present

Volume: 600+ collections
Hours: 900 a.m. - 1:00 a.m. Monday-Friday; closed from
1:00 p.m. to 2:00 p.m.; opens from 2:00 p.m. to 4:30 p.m.

Joseph L. Johnson Papers, physician, educator and college administrator, 1895-date. Biographical information, correspondence, news
articles, reports, minutes, organizational records, 1960-1970.

Ernest Everett Just Papers, zoologist, educator and college administrator, 1883-1941.   Biographical information, reprint articles,
research notes, correspondence, 1910-1940.

Charles Ford Longworthy Papers, chemist and nutritionist, 1864-?

Pete Marshall Murray Papers, physician, educator and hospital
administrator, 1888-1963. Biographical information, correspondence, organizational records, news articles, programs, scrapbooks,
speeches, photographs, certificates and awards, 1910-1970.

Mabel Keaton Staupers Collection, nurse and civil rights activist,
1890-date. Correspondence, biographical information, photographs,
news articles, reports and certificates, 1937-1970.

Daniel Hale Williams Collection, physician, 1856-1931. Biographical information, correspondence, news articles and photographs,
1944-1970.

Louis T. Wright Collection, hospital administrator, physician and
civil rights activist, 1895-1952. Reprints of medical articles by
African American physicians, correspondence, biographical information, organizational records and research statistics, 1878-1952.

George A. Flippin Series, Stewart-Flippin family papers, physician,
?-1929. Correspondence, biographical information memorabilia and
school records, 1852-1974.

FLORIDA

General

University of Miami
Louis Calder Memorial Library
School of Medicine
1601 NW 10th Avenue
Miami, Florida 33101
> Status: permanent
> Update: periodic
> Dated: 1952-present
> Volume: unreported

Medicine in South Florida, 1952 to date. Contains information about refugees and other minority groups. Collection unclassified. Made up of newspaper clippings.

African Americans

Florida State Archives
Bureau of Archives and Record Management
R.A. Gray Building
500 South Bronough Street
Tallahassee, Florida 32399-0250
> Status: permanent
> Update: none
> Dated: 1920-1950
> Volume: 3 cubic feet

Florida State Board of Health. This collection consists of materials from a maternity training program for African Americans. Pamphlets (1930-1955); letters, photographs (1930-1950); and mannequinn (ca. 1945).

Hispanics

Florida State Archives
Bureau of Archives and Record Management
R.A. Gray Building

500 South Bronough Street
Tallahassee, Florida 32399-0250
                    Status: permanent
                    Update: none
                    Dated: 1961-1974
                    Volume: 735 cubic feet

This collection consists of medical, dental, immunization, emergency, and psychiatric, administrative, employee and family medical records. The medical center was set up in the early 1960's to process Cuban refugees entering the US through Miami. This collection has not been processed. Collection open only to medical researchers with approval from Archives' Institutional Review Board.

GEORGIA

General

Medical College of Georgia Library
Augusta, Georgia 30912
                    Status: permanent
                    Update: none
                    Dated: 1836-1860
                    Volume: unreported

Includes materials on the history of medicine in the early 19th and late 18th century; and materials on the Medical College of Georgia. Materials which pertain to minorities include reports on medical cases dealing with patients or with the prevalence of some disease. These reports are found in the Southern Medical Surgical Journal, 1-836-1839 and 1845- 1860.

HAWAII

Pacific Asian Americans

Hawaii State Archives
Iocani Palace Grounds

Honolulu, Hawaii 96813
>Status: permanent
>Update: periodic
>Dated: 1850-1983
>Volume: 25.9 linear feet of fully processed records and approximately 30 cubic feet of records with inventory only.

Department of Health Records. Includes minutes of the Board of Health (1858-1983), records relating to Hansen's Disease (1866-1965) and unprocessed correspondence. Screening by an archivist of records less than 80 years old is required in order to identify and withhold records which may be restricted by statute required prior to granting access.

IDAHO

No Collections Reported

ILLINOIS

African Americans

Illinois State Archives
State Archives Building
Springfield, Illinois 62756
(217)782-4682
>Status: permanent
>Update: none
>Dated: 1940-1963
>Volume: 13 volumes
>Hours: 8:00 - 4:30, Monday-Friday
>8:30 - 3:30, Saturday (except holiday weekends)

No special requirements for consultation of these records.

Commission on Human Relations Minutes of Commission Meetings (RS305.1) 1943-1963, 9 volumes. Minutes discuss attempts to aid African American physicians in establishing practices.

State Commission to Investigate Living Conditions of the Urban
Colored Population/Transcripts of Hearings (RS552.1), 1940-1941,
4 volumes.

INDIANA

No Collections Reported

IOWA

No Collections Reported

KANSAS

Native Americans

Kansas State Historical Society
Manuscripts Department, Center for Historical Research
6425 S.W. 6th Avenue
Topeka, Kansas 66615
913-272-8681
              Status: permanent
              Update: none
              Dated: 1871-1970
              Volume: 73,000+ documents
              Hours: 9:00 a.m. - 4:30 p.m. Monday-Friday
              8:00 - noon Saturdays (except holiday weekends)
Note: Most micro film is available through interlibrary loan.
Materials included in the collection: 89th Congress (1965-1966),
Department of Interior operation of reservations. Ninetieth (90th)
Congress (1967-1970), Department of Interior, Bureau of Indian
Affairs files, letters and memos concerning health care and other
concerns of the Kickapoo and Potawatomi tribes.

Chester Mize was a US representative from Kansas' 2nd district, 1965-1970. The collection includes materials related to the Potawatomi and Kickapoo reservations in Kansas and health care on the reservations.

George Remsburg Papers, 1871-1954. Remsburg was an author, editor, and amateur archeologist. He investigated the Kickapoo Indians of northeast Kansas. Included in the collection is information on consumption among the Kickapoo. Materials in the collection include: letters (1891-1941) and copies of speeches and treaties (1778-1941).

Jotham Meeker was a Baptist minister, Indian Missionary, and printer. The correspondence in the collection relates to his missionary activities and describes the hardships of Indian life, discusses the policy of Indian removal and other national issues affecting Indians, and events at the Ottawa Indian mission. The collection also includes annual reports, expense records, a hand written pamphlet on the Ottawa phonetic system, Meeker's journals, and a manuscript by an Ottawa chief on tribal traditions and ceremonies. Papers, boxes and volumes, also available on microfilm.

John Gill Pratt was a Baptist missionary, teacher, printer, and Indian agent. He came to the Shawnee Baptist Mission in Kansas in 1837. In 1864, he was appointed US agent to the Delawares. The collection includes the personal letters of Pratt, reports to the secretary of the missionary society, sermons, and some records of the Wyandotte, Kansas and Delaware Indian agencies. Papers also available on microfilm, 1834-1899.

KENTUCKY

General

University of Louisville Archives
Louisville, Kentucky 40292
    Status: permanent
    Update: periodic
    Dated: 1920 - 1970

Volume: 50 linear feet

Historical Records of Metro United Way (Louisville). The local United Way and its predecessors go back to 1917. The organization's records seldom refer to minorities, but until 1950, most health and welfare organizations were segregated. Records in this collection are being processed. Those that have been processed include: scrapbooks (1935 - 1970), minutes of health and welfare planning and delivery organizations, multifarious communications and reports reviewing the work of segregated hospitals or social service agencies (1930 - 1970).

African Americans

University of Louisville
Kornhauser Health Sciences Library
Louisville, Kentucky 40292
        Status: permanent
        Update: none
        Dated: 1801-1961
        Volume: 17.75 linear feet
        Hours: 8:00 - 5:00 Monday-Friday
        other times by appointment

WPA Medical Historical Research Project Records 1790 - 1940, Verbatim notes made by a team of federal researchers on a variety of health and medical topics. *Medicine and Its Development in Kentucky* resulted from this project. The WPA Research Materials are typed, verbatim copies of primary and secondary sources (letter, newspaper articles, minutes of health organizations, bulletins, biographical encyclopedias, medical registries, and the like). One series contains biographical information about more than 5,500 physicians, nurses, dentists, hospital administrators, and other assorted health professionals. It is arranged alphabetically by individual names. A number of African American physicians appear here. As with the Caucasian American health professionals, there are transcriptions of oral history interviews containing information probably not published or written anywhere else. Now available on microfilm (32 rolls with guide).

Health Council Records (Louisville), 1926-1961. A predecessor of United Way in Louisville this body considered issues of health and sanitation for the whole community, dealing sometimes with African American institutions and controversies. The record include minutes and correspondence pertaining to the delivery of health care to the African American community in the 1920s. Minutes and correspondence for 1926 and 1927 debate issues such as the need for a African American nursing school and health standards for a African American orphanage and Negro health week observation. .25 linear feet.

Bulletin of the African American Louisville Medical no National College, 1907 - 1908 item no restriction on access to the above material.

University of Louisville Archives
Louisville, Kentucky 40292
            Status: permanent
            Update: periodic
            Dated: 1869 - 1980
            Volume: 130 linear feet

Red Cross Hospital Records, 1907 - 1976. Founded in 1899 by African American physicians, the Red Cross Hospital (later Community Hospital) served Louisville's African American community. The hospital closed in 1975, a victim of desegregation of hospital facilities. Part of the collection is unprocessed. The portion that is processed contains patient records; Houston Baker scrapbooks (1943 - 1951) on director of the Red Cross Hospital; files of Henry Heyburn (1945 - 1974) and Laual Todd Duncan (1857 - 1965) members of the Board of Directors.

Simmons University Records, 1869 - 1971. Simmons University was a African American school that offered a wide range of courses during the late 19th and early 20th centuries. It was affiliated with the National Medical College a medical school for African Americans, during this period and also offered training for nurses and pharmacists. Materials in the collection include: one Simmons Catalogue (1907 - 1908) which covers in depth the Louisville National Medical College and other heath-related programs, photographs (late 1910 -

early 1920), and information on the medical school's founder, Henry Fitzbutler.

University of Louisville President's Office. Records on Louisville Municipal College, 1924 - 1954. Louisville Municipal College was a African American, undergraduate division of the University of Louisville that operated from 1931 until 1951. It offered the B.S. and B.A. degrees. It originated because African American voters were needed to back city bond issues for U of L during the 1920s, which they would not do because African Americans were not admitted to the University. As a compromise, LMC was established in exchange for African American support. Although it operated as a liberal arts college, originally the proposed African American school was supposed to specialize in offering pre-professional training for African Americans who wanted to enter medicine, nursing, dentistry, and other health fields. This plans was abandoned, but the records contain information on it. George C. Wright's 1977 Duke University doctoral dissertation on African Americans in Louisville contains information on the origins of LMC, as well as other aspects of African Americans in the city, including health fields. Materials in the collection include: 25 letters (1920s).

Murray Walls Papers, 1866 - 1980. Murray Walls is the wife of a African American physician who began to practice in the Louisville in 1918. Mrs. Walls' papers contains material on her work as civil rights activists, Dr. Walls medical practice, and the family's involvement in community affairs. Highlights of Dr. Walls' medical career include his graduation from Meharry Medical College in 1917, establishing a practice in Louisville in 1918, joining the Falls City Medical Society, an organization of African American physicians, in the same year, service on the Louisville Health Council in the 1920s, establishment of "well baby clinics" in Louisville's African American community during the 1920s, joining the surgical staff of Red Cross Hospital, a local African American hospital, in 1936, and service on the governing board of Red Cross Hospital from 1942 to 1957.

Murray Walls Papers, 1866 - 1980. Materials in the collection include: correspondence, newspaper clippings, photographs and printed material on Dr. Walls' medical career in Louisville and his leadership in the Louisville Chapter of the NAACP.

Oral History Collection: African American History, 1910-present.
11 individual interviews:

1.   Dr. and Mrs. J.H. Walls. Interviewed in 1973 and 1977.
        The interviews concern the involvement of a prominent
        African American physician and his wife in local civil rights
        issues and medical affairs beginning in the 1910s. It's
        especially good for information on medical practice in the
        African American community; Red Cross Hospital, a African
        American institution; and the Falls City Medical Society, an
        organization of African American physicians. The Walls
        interviews supplement the Walls papers, a description of
        which is included on a separate form. The same goes for the
        interviews on Red Cross Hospital. A description of the Red
        Cross Hospital Records that are in the U of L Archives is on
        a separate form. Generally, these interviews show how
        segregation forced the development of a "society within a
        society." To some extent, middle class African Americans
        had a vested interest in segregation, because it provided a
        built- in market for the goods and services they offered. Red
        Cross Hospital was an example. It closed when other
        hospitals integrated. It should be noted that Louisville City
        Hospital admitted African Americans during this period, but
        they had separate "colored" wards, except for the psychiatric
        ward, which was integrated. Most of the African American
        physicians discussed the integration of the Jefferson County
        Medical Society, which took place in 1953.

2.   Dr. J.B. Bell. Interviewed in 1977. A Louisville African
        American physician discusses the professional limitations
        that were placed upon him because of his race.

3.   Dr. Maurice Rabb. Interviewed in 1977. Rabb grew up in
        Mississippi, attended Fisk University and Meharry Medical
        College, and practiced in Shelbyville, Kentucky, before
        coming to Louisville in 1946. His recollections include
        information on Red Cross Hospital and the Falls City
        Medical Society. He was also concerned with civil rights
        issues. Born c. 1902. Died 1982.

4.   Dr. C. Milton Young, Jr. Interviewed in 1978. A graduate
        of Meharry Medical College and a long-time Louisville

physician discusses medical practice in the African American community and his work with various clinics and health centers. Born c. 1900.

5.   Dr. C. Milton Young, III. Interviewed in 1979. A African American physician discusses his relationship with Red Cross Hospital (see above), the institution's importance to the African American community, and the reasons for its closing. Born 1930.

6.   Dr. Jesse B. Bell. Interviewed in 1979. A Louisville African American physician and former medical director of Red Cross Hospital (see above) discusses his work with the hospital during the 1920s, the integration of Louisville's hospitals, and the reasons for the failure of Red Cross. Born 1904.

7.   Mr. Waverly Johnson. Interviewed in 1979. The administrator of Red Cross Hospital (see above) discusses his role, the problems confronting the institution, and the reasons for its failure.

8.   Rev. Eric Tachau. Interviewed in 1979. A twenty-year member of the board of directors of Red Cross Hospital (see above) describes the work of various administrators, the problems confronting the board, and the reasons for the hospital's failure. A Caucasian American clergyman.

9.   Dr. Albert Goldin. Interviewed in 1979. A Caucasian American physician who served on the board of Red Cross Hospital discusses his role during the institution's last years of existence. Born 1923.

10.   William Summers, III. Interviewed in 1979. Summers served as president of the board of directors of Red Cross Hospital during its last years of existence. He discusses efforts to save the institution.

11.   D.W. Beard. Interviewed in 1979. Beard discusses his twenty years of service on the board of directors of Red Cross Hospital. He covers changes in the character of the

board, divisive issues, and the importance of the institution to the African American community.

LOUISIANA

African Americans

The Historic New Orleans Collection
532 Royal Street
New Orleans, Louisiana 70130
  Status: permanent
  Update: none
  Dated: 1817 - 1871
  Volume: 1410 documents

Cane River Collection. A collection of documents concerning the people of the Cane River area, a community of free people of color. Collection is primarily in French with English summaries available.

New Orleans Public Library
Louisiana Division
219 Loyola Avenue
New Orleans, Louisiana 70140
  Status: permanent
  Update: daily
  Dated: 1769 - present
  Volume; 1,000,000 documents

City Archives Collection. Parts of this collection pertain to the health conditions and/or treatment experienced by minorities. Materials include: New Orleans Health Department. Death certificates kept by the Recorder of Births, Marriages, and Deaths for New Orleans, 1-805-1915. Includes race and place of origin of individual decedents along with cause of death in most cases. These are available on microfilm as are WPA produced annual indexes. The original records are not available for research. Biennial reports, 1898-1928; 1971-1982. Published reports, including statistical tables, some of which contain racial breakdowns.

City Insane Asylum. Records, 1858-1882. Manuscript patient registers showing race and place of origin of individuals committed.

Eye, Ear, Nose and Throat Hospital. Annual reports, 1893-1929 (some missing). Published reports, including statistical tables, some of which contain racial breakdown.

City Smallpox Hospital. Records, 1874- 1879. Manuscript register of patients indicating race and place of origin.

City Cemeteries. Interment records, ca. 1835-1968. Manuscript burial records, most of which include race and place of origin, as well as cause of death, of individuals buried in the various city-owned cemeteries. Also available on microfilm. We also have microfilm copies of the interment records for most of the city's Catholic cemeteries, ca. 1833-1959.

Coroner's Office. Manuscript death records (1905-1979), autopsy records (1844-1979), and insanity (commitment) records (1881-1973), all of which include race and place of origin along with cause of death (or insanity). Also available on microfilm. Insanity records less than 75 years old are not open for research.

Charity Hospital. Admission records (1818-1899) and death registers (1835- 1904). Microfilm copies of the original manuscript records which are not open for research. These include race and place of origin along with the illness and/or cause of death of each individual. This hospital was particularly important to the immigrant population during the nineteenth century.

Newspaper Collection, 1804-present. Our collection is the most extensive for the city of New Orleans. Some of the titles are available only on microfilm. Louisiana News and Louisiana Obituary Indexes should be useful in locating articles relative to minority health care.

Tulane University
Rudolph Matas Medical Library
1430 Tulane Avenue
New Orleans, Louisiana 70712
          Status: permanent
          Update: none

Dated: unreported
Volume: 25 books

Books about history of Native Americans and African Americans.

MAINE

No Collections Reported

MARYLAND

General

National Institute on Aging
Information Center
P.O. Box 8057
Gaithersburg, Maryland 20898
(800)222-2225
Status: permanent
Update: periodic
Dated: 1980-present
Volume: unreported

Age Page: Minorities and how they grow old. One page fact sheet intended for a lay audience.

White House Conference on Aging: Aging and Minorities, Leaflet intended for a general audience on topics of concern to the minority elderly and their families.

Profile of America's Elderly: Racial and Ethnic Diversity of America's Elderly Population. 1993.

Profile of America's Elderly: Living Arrangements of the Elderly. 1993.

African Americans

The Johns Hopkins Medical Institution
Alan Mason Chesney Medical Archives
2024 East Monument Street
Suite 1-500
Baltimore, Maryland 21205
(410)955-5043
        Status: permanent
        Update: periodic
        Dated: 1893-1923
        Volume: 13 books, 6 boxes of documents

The Johns Hopkins Hospital Committee on the Colored Orphan Asylum, 1898-1912. 1 volume.

The Johns Hopkins Convalescent Home patient registry, 1914-1917. 1 volume.

Eleven petty cash books.

Five books of financial invoices.

One box of material regarding by-laws and history of the Johns Hopkins Hospital Committee on the Colored Orphan Asylum. This box contains the names of patients discharged from the Johns Hopkins Hospital Colored Orphan Asylum during a few specific years.

The Johns Hopkins Hospital Trustee minutes. These include material regarding the Johns Hopkins Hospital Colored Orphan Asylum. 3 volume.

National Cancer Institute
Building 31, Room 10A18
Bethesda, Maryland 20205
        Status: permanent
        Update: periodic
        Dated: 1980-present
        Volume: 5-10 pamphlets ?
Description: Office of Cancer Communications

What Black Americans should know about Cancer. This pamphlet explains the rates and risks of cancer among African Americans and answers the most-often asked questions on cancer; its causes, detection, prevention, treatment, rehabilitation and common misconceptions. Publication is available free of charge from the above address.

National Heart, Lung, and Blood Institute
Publications Section
Bethesda, Maryland 20205
> Status: permanent
> Update: periodic
> Dated: 1975-present
> Volume: unreported

1.   *Adolescents with Sickle Cell Anemia and Sickle Cell Trait.* This brochure is designed to help the adolescent who has sickle cell trait or anemia understand the condition.

2.   *A Bibliography: Comprehensive Sickle Cell Centers.* Presents bibliographic references of significant publications from the Comprehensive Sickle Cell Centers during 1972-80. Serves as a source of information and study findings related to sickle cell disease.

3.   *African Americans and High Blood Pressure.* Describes what high blood pressure is, its importance to African Americans, the need for treatment, and the role of the patient's family.

4.   *Directory of National, Federal, and Local Sickle Cell Disease Programs.* Listing includes comprehensive sickle cell centers, sickle cell screening and education clinics, national centers for family planning services, VA hospitals, state health departments, and public and private organizations.

5.   *Final Report of the National Black Health Providers Task Force on High Blood Pressure Education and Control.* Action-oriented document for health care providers and

others who participate in the control of high blood pressure among .

6.   *Review and Response to the Final Report of the National Black Health Providers Task Force on High Blood Pressure Education and Control.* The NHLBI looks at each of the task force recommendations individually, and indicates what steps can be taken to meet them.

7.   *Sickle Cell Fundamentals.* Describes the difference between sickle cell trait and sickle cell anemia, the clinical features of sickle cell anemia, laboratory diagnosis and treatment. Information concerning the molecular basis of the disease, inheritance factors, geographic distribution and a glossary are included in this illustrated booklet.

8.   *Your Employee with Sickle Cell.* Provides a brief overview of sickle cell anemia and sickle cell trait and explains what an employer can expect from someone who has either. Encourages employers to hire individuals who have the trait or disease.

MASSACHUSETTS

African Americans

Boston University
Mugar Memorial Library
Nursing Archives, Special Collections
771 Commonwealth Avenue
Boston, Massachusetts 02215
            Status: permanent
            Update: periodic
            Dated: 1922-1979 (Present ?)
            Volume: unreported

American Nurses Association. The collection contains letters and minutes of the ANA Joint Committee with the National Association of Colored Graduate Nurses (1928-1950), reprints of articles about minorities in nursing, Mary Ellen Mchoney, and African American patients. This collection also contains two reprints of articles about nursing schools by M. Elizabeth Carnegie.

M. Elizabeth Carnegie, Nurse. A leader in public health nursing, tuberculosis control, women in Africa and nursing research. Former dean of the Florida A & M College School of Nursing, former Director of the Hampton Institute School of Nursing. Formerly on the editorial staff of the American Journal of Nursing and currently on the editorial staff of *Nursing Outlook*. One manuscript book composed of articles (1960-1976), letter (1975), photographs and speeches (1944-1975).

Eva M. Noles, Nurse, 1956-1979. Leader in nursing - nursing of the patient with cancer - public health nursing. She was Director of Nursing at Roswell Park Memorial Institute (1945-1974). Articles (1971-1979), letters (1971-1979), newspaper clippings (1974), speeches (1970-1975), and certificates (1964-1973).

Radcliffe College
Schlesinger Library
10 Garden Street
Cambridge, Massachusetts 02138
     Status: permanent
     Update: updated (upon receipt of information)
     Dated: 1880-1870's to present
     Volume: unreported

Black Women Oral History Project, A collection of 72 oral histories, of which 9 were with women in health-related fields.

1.   May Chinn, 1896-1980. General Medicine and Cancer. Oral history transcript.

2.   Florence Edmonds, 1890-1983 Public Health Nurse. Oral history transcript, photographs, and clippings.

3.   Lena Edwards, 1900-1986 Gynecology and Obstetrics. Oral history transcript, clippings, and photographs.

4.   Dorothy Ferebee, 1898-1980. Obstetrics and Preventive Medicine. Oral history transcript, photographs, clippings, and pamphlets.

5.   Flemmie Kittrell, 1904-1980. Nutrition. Oral history transcript, photographs, and articles.

6.   Eunice Laurie, 1899-? Public Health nurse. Oral history transcript and photographs.

7.   Mabel Staupers, 1890-? Nursing. Videotape.

8.   Ruth Temple, 1892 - 1984 Preventive Medicine and Public Health. Oral history transcript, photographs, and clippings.

9.   Mary Thompson, 1902-1985 Dentistry. Oral history transcript, photographs, and clippings.

Native Americans

Boston University
Mugar Memorial Library
Nursing Archives, Special Collections
771 Commonwealth Avenue
Boston, Massachusetts 02215
          Status: permanent
          Update: periodic
          Dated: 1922-1979 (Present ?)
          Volume: unreported

Elinor D. Gregg, Nurse, 1922-1953. Supervisor of Public Health Nursing in the Bureau of Indian Affairs, 1924-1939. This collection contains her notebook of places visited and reports, correspondence, and various rules and regulations for nurses and inspectors of the Indian Services. Letters (1924- 1967), articles (1922-1949), newspaper clippings, reports (1922-1932), photographs, notes on research and field trips and administrative notes.

MICHIGAN

General

University of Michigan School of Nursing Correspondence, 1925. Discusses racial discrimination in the nursing home.

Midwest Migrant Health Information Office. Organization established to improve the health and living conditions of migrant farmworkers in six states of upper midwest. 1962-1991. Five linear feet.

African Americans

University of Michigan
Bentley Historical Library
1150 Beal Avenue
Ann Arbor, Michigan 48109
          Status: permanent
          Update: annual
          Dated: 1866-1930
          Volume: unreported

Margaret Bell, 1888-1969. Bell Papers, 1919-1956. Chairman of the Department of Physical Education for women of the University of Michigan and physician in the University Health Service. Six linear feet.

Margaret Bell, 1888-1969. Bell Photograph Series, 1920-1960. .7 linear feet.

Summit Medical Center, Ann Arbor, Michigan. Summit Medical Center Photograph Series, 1969-1976. One folder.

Detroit Urban League Records. Photographs, motion pictures, league conferences and Green Pastures Camp. Departmental files relating to community services, housing, health and welfare, job development, employment, and education. 96 linear feet, 1 oversized folder. 1916-present.

Remus Grant Robinson Papers, Physician and Civic leader, 1904-1970. Contains student notes and other materials taken while attending the University of Michigan Medical School, 1927-1930.

Native Americans

University of Michigan
Bentley Historical Library
1150 Beal Avenue
Ann Arbor, Michigan 48109
      Status: permanent
      Update: annual
      Dated: 1866-1930
      Volume: unreported

"Variola" by Noah Bates. Thesis, 1866. Contains an account of a small pox epidemic among the Indians on a reservation in Brant County, Ontario.

MINNESOTA

No Collections Reported

MISSISSIPPI

General

American Nurses' Association
420 Pershing Road
Kansas City, Missouri 64108
      Status: permanent
      Update: periodic
      Dated: 1961-present
      Volume: unreported

The American Nurses' Association publishes a selected bibliography on minority groups in nursing. These articles mainly deal with minorities in the health professions but several notations concern articles which provide historical perspectives.

Additionally, ANA is publishing *Contemporary Minority Leaders in Nursing: Afro-American, Hispanic and Native American Perspectives.*

African Americans

State of Mississippi
Department of Archives and History
P.O. Box 571
Jackson, Mississippi 39205
    Status: permanent
    Update: none
    Dated: 1931-1935
    Volume: unreported

Afro-American Hospital Records, 1931- 1935. The Afro-American Hospital of Yazoo City was established in 1928 as an exclusively African American owner/African American operated hospital. The collection contains one- patient register providing information on patients, including admitting diagnosing, discharge diagnosing and related information. The original volume is restricted from use until January 1, 2006. Microfilm of the patient register contains all information except patients names and other identifying information.

Panther Burn Plantation account books. Time frame 1859-1862; 1864-1865; 1879; 1881-1883. Two volumes.

Washington University
School of Medicine
The Bernard Becker Medical Library
Archives and Rare Book Section
660 S. Euclid Avenue
St. Louis, Missouri 63110
(314)362-4239
    Status: permanent
    Update: irregular
    Dated: 1895-1980
    Volume: 105.5 (out of total Archival holdings of 2300) feet

Robert E. Shank papers, 1946-1980, 84 feet Includes correspondence, reports, documents, architectural plans, manuscripts, speeches, and conference proceedings. This material documents Dr. Shank's interest in nutrition, diet, rehabilitation, hospital administration, preventive medicine and public health.

Robert J. Terry papers, 1895-1966, 12 fee Includes correspondence, manuscripts, scrapbooks, card files, certificates, pamphlets and reprints of articles. This material documents Dr. Terry's interest in anatomy, anthropology and eugenics.

Mildred Trotter Papers, 1922-1976, 3.5 feet includes correspondence, reports, documents and manuscripts. The papers document Dr. Trotter's research on the hair, the skeleton, and race.

Park J. White Papers, 1913-1979, 6 feet includes correspondence, lectures, speeches, manuscripts, notes, reports, certificates and photographs. The material documents Dr. White's interest in pediatrics, hospital administration, public health and race relations.

Oral Histories: Robert E. Shank 1980
                   Mildred Trotter 1972
                   Park J. White 1979
                   Washington University Medical Center
                   Desgregration History Project, 1990.

MONTANA

Native Americans

Montana Historical Society
225 North Roberts Street
Helena, Montana 59601
(406)444-2694
         Status: permanent
         Update: periodic
         Dated: 1812-1977
                   Volume: unreported

Blackfeet Indian Agency Records, 1941- 1942. (SC 907) Report of Dr. H. F. Schrader concerning the Blackfeet Indian Reservation health problems. 14 p.p.

Flathead Indian Agency Records, 1864- 1968. (SC 885) Correspondence from Indian Agent, Charles Hutchins to Territorial Governor. Includes letter from physician Charles Shaft reporting tribal health conditions. 1 p.

State Board of Health, 1908-1977 (RS 28). Correspondence and reports. Health conditions on Indian reservations are found in subject files. (2 feet)

Journal of William Fraser Tolmie, Physician and fur trader, 1812-1886.

Grimes, Clinton E. Alcoholism and Montana Indian people: toward an off-reservation solution: a study (written by) Clint Grimes, prepared by the Montana United Indian Association for, and under a grant, from the Additive Diseases Bureau of the Montant State Department of Institutions. Helena Mont.: The Association, (1975). 45 leaves; 28 cm.

Urban Management Consultants of San Franscisco, Inc. Profile of the Montana Native American, prepared for Coordinator of Indian Affairs by Urban Management Connsultants of San Franscisco, Inc. San Fransciso: The Company, 1974. 247 p., charts, 28 cm.
Svingen, Orland J. The administrative history of the Northern Cheyenne Indian Reservation, 1877-1900 (microform), by Orlan Jerome Svinge. 1982.

NEBRASKA

Native Americans

Nebraska State Historical Society
P.O. Box 82554
1500 R Street
Lincoln, Nebraska 68501

(402)471-4751
(402)471-3100 fax
    Status: permanent
    Update: none
    Dated: 1859-1970
    Volume: 41 articles

LaFlesche Family, 1859-1939, Picotte Papers 1885-1917. Collection
contains papers of Dr. Susan LaFlesche Picotte, the first American
Indian woman to become a doctor of medicine. She became a
physician to the Omaha Indians where she campaigned for better
health care. Materials include: correspondence (1885-1917), diary
(1910- 1911) and reports.

Joseph Armitage Paxson Diary, 1869-1870. Collection consists of
a diary kept by Dr. Paxson while serving as a physician to the
Winnebago Indians (original diary located in the Wisconsin Historical
Society).

NEVADA

No Collections Reported

NEW HAMPSHIRE

No Collections Reported

NEW JERSEY

General

University of Medicine and Dentistry
Georgie R. Smith Library - Archives
100 Bergen Street
Newark, New Jersey 07103
    Status: permanent

Update: periodic
Dated: 1954-present
Volume: unreported

David Opdyke Collection, 1954-1981. Dr. Opdyke was Chairman of the Acceptance Committee. He established a program titled Students for Medicine which works with minority undergraduate students who are interested in a career in medicine or dentistry. 10 letters, 1970s and 1 oral history transcription, 1956-1981.

Oral History Program, in progress. Interviews with minority faculty members.

NEW MEXICO

No Collections Reported

NEW YORK

African Americans

Schomburg Center for Research in Black Culture
The New York Public Library
515 Malcolm X Boulevard
New York, New York 10037
        Status: permanent
        Update: none
        Dated: 1908-1958
        Volume: 4 linear feet

May Edward Chinn Papers, 1926-1980. General Medicine and Cancer detection among African Americans. Collection includes certificates, letters and personal and family papers.

Lafargue Clinic Records, 1946-1958. Records of a low-cost mental health clinic established in the basement of St. Philips Episcopal

Church in Harlem. Contains letters, articles, case files, newspaper clippings, clinic and personnel records.

National Association of Colored Graduate Nurses, 1908-1952. Minutes, correspondence, memoranda, reports, scrapbooks, and printed material of an organization founded in 1908 to achieve higher professional standards; to break down discrimination in nursing profession; and to develop leadership among African Americans nurses.

Jewel Plummer Cobb Papers, 1944-1990 (bulk 1960-1990). Educator, college administrator and biologist specializing in cancer research, Dr. Cobb is known for her work in cell morphology, her promotion of the advancement of women in scientific fields, and her activities on behalf of minorities in the profession. Collection consists of grant proposals, reports, laboratory and other notes, manuscripts and published articles documenting Cobb's research on melanoma. In addition, there are texts of her speeches, and minutes and reports for the Committee on Minorities and Women in Science of the National Science Foundation, 1975-1980.

Leonidas H. Berry Papers, 1932-1988. The papers document the medical career of Berry, a gastroenterologist. Collection concists of personal and professional papers, writings pertaining to his profession, and contributions of African Americans in medicine. Included is information regarding an A.M.E. Church health program he helped to establish in the 1960s, and Berry's files for the National Medical Association.

Lincoln School for Nurses Collection, 1840-1987. Founded in 1898 to provide nursing education for African American women when such training was not available elsewhere. The first graduating class was in 1900, and the last was in 1961. A total of 1,864 African American women from the U.S. and abroad attended Lincoln. The collection consists of annual reports, anniversary booklets, and news bulletins. Material from 1840-1898 documents the Society for the Relief of Worthy, Aged, Indigent Colored Person which operated on the site occupied by the Lincoln School. Included are annual reports for the Lincoln Hospital and Home, where the nurses received clinical experience.

Medical Committee for Human Rights, 1964-66. Records of organization established by the Council of Freedom Organizations to recruit health care personnel and provide medical care for civil rights workers who participated in the Mississippi Freedom Summer Project and for local African American residents. Includes correspondence, reports, memoranda, minutes, financial records, membership and fundraising files, committee files, material from local chapters and printed literature.

Sylvester Carter Papers, 1930-82. Hand surgeon. Collection consists of letters, writings, certificates, programs of professional conferences attended by and participated in by Carter, photographs and other materials dealing with his professional activities. Also included are thousands of slides of hand operations performed by Carter.

New York Hospital-Cornell Medical Center
Medical Archives
1300 York Avenue
New York, New York 10021
     Status: permanent
     Update: periodic
     Dated: 1951-1974
     Volume: 20 linear inches

Children's Blood Foundations, Inc., 1951- 1974. This organization cared for children with Thalessemia, Sickle Cell anemia and other genetic blood disorders. Materials include pamphlets, reports and photographs.

Native Americans

New York Hospital-Cornell Medical Center
Medical Archives
1300 York Avenue
New York, New York 10021
     Status: permanent
     Update: none
     Dated: 1953-1981
     Volume: 34 linear inches

Papers of Muriel Carbery, Navaho Field Project Series, 1955-1961. Program of Cornell Medical College and School of Nursing to bring health care and training to Navaho communities centered in Many Farms, Arizona. Materials include books, pamphlets, letters, articles, newspaper clippings, reports, and photographs.

Papers of Dr. Carl Muschenheim, 1966- 1977. Dr. Muschenheim was concerned with treatment of native Americans and Eskimos for primarily pulmonary disease and tuberculosis. Materials include Letters (1966-1977), newspaper clippings, map (1956), and reports.

Papers of Dr. Wash McDermott, 1953-1981. A small portion of Dr. McDermott's papers deal with his involvement with Cornell Navaho Field Health Projects. Dr. McDermott was Professor of Public Health who also worked on Community Projects involving African American, Hispanic and Asian American peoples. The collection is not fully processed but known materials include letters, oral history (1972), newspaper clippings, and reports.

Cornell University Medical College - Navaho - Cornell Field Health Project, 1955-1961. Program to bring health care and attach health care to Navaho communities. Materials include pamphlets, letters, articles, photographs, minutes and reports.

NORTH CAROLINA

General

Wake Forest University
Dorothy Carpenter Medical Archives
Bowman Gray School of Medicine
Medical Center Boulevard
Winston-Salem, North Carolina 27157
(910)716-3690
      Status: permanent
      Update: none
      Dated: mid 19th century - present
      Volume: 1,173 cubic feet

Processed and catalogoued collections on the history and development of the Medical School and its relationship with North Carolina Baptist Hospital. This history parallels and includes the development of health care for minority populations in the surrounding counties.

NORTH DAKOTA

No Collections Reported

OHIO

General

Ohio Historical Society State Archives
1982 Velma Avenue
Columbus, Ohio 43202
        Status: permanent
        Update: periodic
        Dated: 1820-1978
        Volume: unreported

The State Archives contains many records on medical or health information of individuals, with race, ethnic group identification as descriptive information. Those records which contain this identifier include: Athens Mental Health Center, 1875-1925; Boys' Industrial School, 1860-1955; Cleveland State Hospital, 1855-1972; Columbus State Hospital, 1840-1978; Columbus State Institution, 1874-1970; Dayton Mental Health Center, 1852-1955; Gallipolis State Institution, 1890-1960; Girls' Industrial School, 1860-1935; London Correctional Institution, 1915- 1955; Longview State Hospital, 1852-1951; Madison Home, 1885-1948; Massillon State Hospital, 1885-1940; Ohio Penitentiary, 1820-1970; Ohio Reformatory for Women, 1915-1965; Ohio School for the Deaf, 1830-1930; Ohio Soldiers and Sailors Home, 1885-1930; Ohio State Sanatorium, 1905-1930; Ohio Veterans Orphan's Home, 1870-1902; State School for the Blind, 1870-1935; Toledo Mental Health Center, 1880-1970; Ohio Department of Health, Division of Vital Statistics, Tabulations of Death, 1920-1967, State of Ohio Death Certificates, 1908-1936; Ohio Industrial Commission, Daily Record of Proceedings, 1912-1974; Ohio State Liability, Board of Awards, Appearance Docket, 1912-1913.

African Americans

Bowling Green State University
Women's Studies Archives
Bowling Green, Ohio 43403
Center for Archive Collections (between 1st and 2nd line)
Hours: 8:30a.m. - 4:30 p.m. (opened additional hours during school year)
        Status: permanent
        Update: collection complete
        Dated: 1920-1981
        Volume: 5 linear feet

Ella P. Stewart Collection, 1920-1981. Ella Stewart was the first African American woman to graduate from the University of Pittsburg School of Pharmacology. The collection is composed of her scrapbooks illustrating her full and active life.

Cleveland Health Sciences Library
Historical Division
11000 Euclid Avenue
Cleveland, Ohio 44106
        Status: permanent
        Update: none
        Dated: 1922-1978
        Volume: 5 linear feet

Forest City Hospital Archives, 1922-1978. This hospital was founded by African Americans and was intended to be the first interracial hospital in Cleveland. Contents of the collection includes pamphlets, letters, articles, newspaper clippings, oral histories, minutes and pictures.

Archives and Special Collections
Rembert E. Stokes Learning Resources Center Library
Wilberforce University

Wilberforce, Ohio 45384-1003
    Status: permanent
    Update: none
    Dated: 1914
    Volume: one document

Steward, S. Maria, Physician. Dr. Steward was a African American physician who taught at Wilberforce University in the early 1900s. Collection contains one paper presented on August 11, 1914, titled Women in Medicine.

OKLAHOMA

American Indian

Chickasaw Council House Museum
Capital Reserve
P.O. Box 717
Tishomingo, Oklahoma 73460
    Status: permanent
    Update: periodic
    Dated: 1540-1920
    Volume: unreported

Chickasaw Cultural Materials. The collection pertains to the Chickasaw Indians. Their culture through the years up to 1920. Including medical, dental and pharmaceutical records. Collection includes books, letters, cassettes, microfilm, photographs and newspaper clippings.

University of Oklahoma
Health Sciences Center Library
1000 Stanton Young Drive
P.O. Box 26901
Oklahoma City, Oklahoma 73190
    Status: permanent
    Update: annual
    Dated: 1876-present
    Volume: 50,000+ documents

OREGON

No Collections Reported

PENNSYLVANIA

General

Medical College of Pennsylvania
Archives and Special Collections
3300 Henry Avenue
Philadelphia, Pennsylvania 19129
          Status: permanent
          Update: monthly
          Dated: 1850-present
          Volume: unreported

Archives and Special Collections on Women in Medicine. A collection
relating to women physicians in the 19th and 20th centuries consisting
of over 200 books and theses, over 4500 reprints, and over 2000
photographs. This collection as it relates to minorities includes: *Books*:
Dubois, W.E.B. *The Philadelphia Negro: A Social Study*, 1899. Green,
Norma Kidd. *Iron Eye Family: The Children of Joseph LaFlesche*,
1969. Andrews, Lynn V. *Medicine Woman*, 1981.

Jones, David E. *Sanapia: Comanche Medicine Woman*, 1972.
contributions of African American Women to America, Vol. I & II.
ed, Mauianna W. Davis, Ed.D. Pamphlets: Alpha Kappa Alpha
Sorority, Inc. *"Women in Dentistry,"* 1971 (2 copies) Cassette Tapes:
Oral histories recorded in 1978 Brown, Dorothy L. (1919-) Nichols,
Victoria (1944-) Spurlock, Jeanne (1921-) Manuscripts: Two separate
introductions of Helen O. Dickens, M.D. by Emily H. Mudd, Ph.D.,
(1970 and 1978) *Photocopy of a Paper* presented at South Carolina's
First Intern Women's Year Conference. *Women in the Medical
Profession in South Carolina* by Sophire W. Wilson. 1 article by
Margaret Jerrido which was printed in the *Alumnae News*, spring 1979.
The collection also contains correspondence between the former
librarian, Ida Draeger and African American alumnae, and lists of
African American women graduates which were periodically updated
and reprinted.

African Americans

Pennsylvania Historial and Museum Collection
William Penn Memorial Museum and Archives Building
Box 1026
Harrisburg, Pennsylvania 17108-1026
(717)787-3384
      Status: permanent
      Update: periodic
      Dated: 1899-present
      Volume: unreported

Harry Shapiro Collection, 1956-59. Records of Harry Shapiro, Philadelphian, Republican senator in the Pennsylvania legislature, 1933-44, secretary of the Pennsylvania's Department of Welfare, 1955-58, and secretary of the Commonwealth's Department of Public Welfare, 1958-59. Included are materials concerning the Department of Welfare (reports and recommendations, 1956 and 1959; statistics, 1959.

Commonwealth of Pennsylvania. Mental Health Center. Philadelphia Region. Conjoint Mental Health Board. Minutes and reports, 1956-57.

Commonwealth of Pennsylvania. Mental Health Center. Research and Statistics Unit. Monthly reports, 1957.

Commonwealth of Pennsylvania. Department of Public Health. Office of Public Assistance. Statistics, 1959.

William A. Stone Papers, 1893-1903. William Alexis Stone (1846-1920) was a soldier in the Civil War, a district attorney in Tioga County, a U.S. Attorney for the Western District of Pennsylvania, a member of the 52nd, 53rd, 54th, and 55th Congresses, and was Governor from 1899 to 1903.

Legislation Files, 1899-1902 contain: lists of appropriations to such State-aided institutions as the Frederick Douglass Memorial Hospital and Nursing School in Philadelphia, the Aged and Infirm Colored Women's Home in Pittsburgh, and the Home for Colored Children in Allegheny City.

Reports File, 1899-1903 contains the Board of Public Charities, 1901-02, with much the same information in the Preliminary Report for 1900.

Records of the Department of Health. Charged with the responsibility of protecting the health of the citizens of the Commonwealth, the Department of Health enforces statutes and relations pertaining to public health matters, and works to insure the prevention and suppression of disease. The Department was created in 1905 to replace the State Board of Health and Vital Statistics which had been established in 1885. Specific agency duties include the areas of drug and narcotics control, maternal and child health programs, dental health, crippled childred services, health education, preventive health programs, and comprehensive health planning.

Bureau of Sanitary Engineering. Sanitary Engineer Epidemic Reports, 1917. Discusses typhoid fever on the farms of William Jones and Samuel Ruth of East Fallowfield Township, Chester County, Ercildtown, PA, about four miles from Coatesville, PA. The two farms were adjoining owned by the families of William Jones and Samuel Ruth, both families African American.

Native Americans

Commonwealth of Pennsylvania State Archives
Box 1026
Harrisburg, Pennsylvania 17108-1026
          Status: permanent
          Update: none
          Dated: 1972
          Volume: unreported

Folk Medicine of the Delaware and related Algankian Indians. By Gladys Tantaqudgeon, Harrisonburg: Pennsylvania Historical and Museum Commission, 1972.

RHODE ISLAND

Native Americans

Rhode Island State Archives
Room 43 State House
Providence, RI 02903
>Status: permanent
>Update: none
>Dated: 1735-1842
>Volume: 200 pages

SOUTH CAROLINA

General

South Carolina Archives
1430 Senate Street
P.O. Box 11669
Columbia, South Carolina 29211
>Status: permanent
>Update: annual
>Dated: 1850-1880
>Volume: unreported

Contains information regarding health and medical treatment of minorities.

Mortality schedules of the Federal Census, 1850-1880.

Petitions of physicians who attended prisoners of the Vasey rebellion.

Charters of minority health care corporations.

Records of the Freedman's Bureau.

African Americans

Medical University of South Carolina
Waring Historical Library
171 Ashley Avenue

Charleston, South Carolina
Hours: 8:30 a.m. - 5:00 p.m.
       Status: permanent
       Update: annual
       Dated: 1822-1981
       Volume: 24 documents
Information on ethic minorities dispersed in general collection: 20 books, (1848-1981) and 6 theses or inaugural dissertations relating to slave health, 1822-1856.

Lucy Hughes Brown, Physician, -1911. Biographical material and photograph.

Matilda Arabelle Evans, Physician, -1935. Biographical material and photograph.

Anna DeCosta Banks, Nurse, 1869-1930. Biographical material and photograph.

Alonzo Clifton McClennan, Physician, 1855-1912. Biographical material.

Hospital and Training School for Nurses, organized 1893. A hospital and nursing school for African Americans. Historical notes, several issues of *Hospital Herald*, the hospital's journal and the nursing school's graduation programs and photographs.

McClennan-Banks Memorial Hospital 1959- 1977. An out growth of the hospital and nursing school. Materials include historical notes.

Palmetto Medical, Dental and Pharmaceutical Association, 1896. A professional society for African Americans. Materials include historical notes.

SOUTH DAKOTA

Native Americans

University of South Dakota
School of Medicine

Division of Surgery
2501 W. 22nd Street
Sioux Falls, South Dakota 57105
    Status: permanent
    Update: periodic
    Dated: 800-present
    Volume: 45-50 documents

John B. Gregg, M.D. personal publications. Research work relating to health problems in the Native Americans who live in the South Dakota region began in almost 1955 and is still ongoing. Included are reports relating to health problems as they exist now and investigation into health problems that have existed in this region during the pasts millennium, as they appear in human remains and artifacts.

TENNESSEE

African Americans

Tennessee State Library and Archives
403 Seventh Avenue North
Nashville, Tennessee 37243-0312
    Status: permanent
    Update: periodic
    Dated: 1780-1970
    Volume: unreported
    Hours: 8:00 a.m. - 6:00 p.m. Monday-Saturday
The archives contain several collections describing plantation and slave life. Recounts about health and health services might appear in these collections. Collection where specific health concerns are mentioned include:

Esther G. Wright Boyd Memoir, 1840-1860. These memoirs were written at the request of Dr. Walter L. Fleming, son-in-law of Mrs. Boyd. They deal with conditions and social customs in the Parish of Rapides, Louisiana, in the period preceding the Civil War. Mrs. Boyd wrote of family life, schools, churches and social life.

James Green Carson Family Papers, 1835-1849. Catherine (Waller) Carson's letter of January 26, 1836, tells about life at "Cane Brake" one of her husband's plantations near Natchez, Mississippi. In addition to describing her house, she writes about the slaves and their relations with the white family. Her husband's letter of June 14, 1849, tells about a cholera epidemic which has caused the deaths of slaves on his and neighboring plantations and describes several remedies for the disease.

Christopher Hutchings Papers, 1804-1970. Businessman and Planter, Madison County Tennessee. These papers include account bills, notes, receipts, correspondence, genealogical data, legal documents, medical accounts, plantation records, school records and some miscellaneous items.

Lawrence Family Papers, 1780-1944. Correspondence, diaries, documents, genealogical data, military papers, poems, scrapbook of newspaper clippings, and an autobiography of Emily (Donelson) Boddie Walton, relating to members of the Lawrence family of Nashville, Tennessee. Includes material on family life before and after the Civil War in and near Nashville, farming, life on "Angola", a Louisiana plantation, practice of medicine, trips to New Orleans, New York, Newport, R.E., and abroad and William Pitt Lawrence's service as surgeon for the 3rd Regt., Tennessee Militia, War of 1812. Members of the family presented include Dr. William Pitt Lawrence (1784-1853), his wife, Nancy Pomeroy (Risley) Lawrence, their son, William Luther Bigelow Lawrence (1828-1902), farmer and lawyer of Nashville, his wife, Corinne (Hayes) Lawrence, and his wife's sister Adelicia (Hayes) Franklin Acklen Cheatham.

Harry S. Mustard, Photograph album, 1925-1930. Consists of photgraphs taken of children, buildings, and events during Dr. Harry S. Mustard's five-year work with the Commonwealth Fund in Rutherford County, Tennessee. One volume.

Fisk University Library
Special Collections
Nashville, Tennessee 37203
        Status: permanent
        Update: periodic
        Dated: 1893-present

Volume: unreported
Materials relating to African American health, physicians, medical history, gerontology, etc., are interspersed within the various special collections.

Papers of Robert Tecumsec Burt 1873-1955 (Papers 1893-1972). Five manuscript boxes of Clarksville, Tennessee physician and Meharry graduate.

Rosenwald Collection, 1917-1948 (Archives) Letters for financial support for African American hospitals, nursing programs; also includes items on Tuskegee syphilis project.

Oral history interviews with the following physicians:
1.   Dr. Dorothy Brown, Surgeon
2.   Dr. Mae Carroll, Physician
3.   Dr. Jimmie Logan, Ophthalmologist
4.   Dr. Montague Cobb, Anatomist
5.   Dr. Edward Perry Crump, Pediatrician
6.   Dr. Jeanne Spurlock, Child Psychiatrist
7.   Dr. Doris Wright, Pediatrician
8.   Dr. Matther Walker, Surgeon
9.   Dr. Elizabeth Backus, Obstetrician

Meharry Medical College Library
1005 D.B. Todd Boulevard
Kresge Learning Resources Center
3rd Floor-Library
Nashville, Tennessee 37208
        Status: permanent
        Update: Continually
        Dated: 1876 - Present
        Volume: Storage boxes: 701
        Document Boxes: 352
        File Cabinets: 48
        Books: 46 shelves
        Videss, Cassettes, and Pictures: 275
        Collections: 30 processed and unprocessed

Black Medical History Collection, 1800-Present. Collection includes books, videos, letters, pictures, articles, and newspaper clippings.

Evelyn K. Tomes Collection: A Living History of Black American Nurses, (Late 1800's to present). Collection includes books, videos, manuscript collections of early African American nurses. Fifteen video tapes of early African American nurses; pictures of early deans of the MMC Nursing School; Bronze plaques with engraved names of all nursing graduates of the MMC Nursing School; Books on the history of nursing, including histories of African Americans in nursing; and, cassette tapes of early nurses.

University of Tennessee
Center for Health Sciences
800 Madison Avenue
Memphis, Tennessee 38163
            Status: permanent
            Update: annual
            Dated: 1910-1970
            Volume: 64 documents

Sickle Cell Collection, 1910-1970 This collection comprises 64 bound volumes of article reprints on sickle cell disease. Dr. L.W. Diggs developed and continually updates this collection with recent articles.

TEXAS

General

Harris County Medical Archive
Houston Academy of Medicine
Texas Medical Center Library
1133 M.D. Anderson Boulevard
Houston, Texas 77030
(713)795-4200
            Status: permanent
            Update: monthly
            Dated: 1920-1980
            Volume: 3000 cubic feet
The archive collects all materials related to health care, biomedical research and medical education; and many of the collections contain material related to the contributions of minorities. Identifies and

separated materials include: 10 books, 1940-date; 200 newspaper clippings, 1965-date; 150 photographs 1940-date.

Houston Metropolitan Research Center
Houston Public Library
500 McKinney Street
Houston Texas, 77002
     Status: permanent
     Update: periodic
     Dated: unreported
     Volume: unreported
The library contains various items in different unprocessed and processed collections which pertain to family medical history and health considerations of Houston's African American and Mexican American communities. Two such collections are:

The Houston Mexican American Archival Collection

The Houston Afro-American Archival Collection

University of Texas
Health Science Center at Dallas Library
5323 Harris Hines Boulevard
Dallas, Texas 75235
     Status: permanent
     Update: monthly
     Dated: unknown
     Volume: 108 documents

History of the Health Sciences. Several monographs and journal articles concerning health care to minorities are included, but not identified separately, in the History of Health Sciences collection.

University of Texas
Health Sciences Center at San Antonio Archives
703 Floyd Curl Drive
San Antonia, Texas 78284
     Status: permanent
     Update: none
     Dated: 1976-1982
     Volume: unreported

Camino Real Health Systems Agency Papers, 1976-1982. Records of an organization designed to coordinate health care services to minorities and the poor, minutes publications and other administrative records.

University of Texas, Medical Branch
Moody Medical Library
Blocker History of Medicine Collection
Galveston, Texas 77550-2774
          Status: permanent
          Update: periodic
          Dated: 1953-1973
          Volume: 2 document

University of Texas Medical Branch, Alumni Association Records, 1953-1973. Materials concerning minority students includes one folder of two documents.

African Americans

Texas State Library
Lorenzo De Zavala State Archives and Library Building
Box 12927
Austin, Texas 78711
          Status: permanent
          Update: annual
          Dated: 1937-1946
          Volume: unreported
          Hours: 8:00 a.m. - 5:00 p.m. Monday
The Texas State Library has records from the Department of Health. Specific items in these records are: Negro Programs, 1941-1946 (includes - Negro College Health Programs, Bishop College Medical and Dental Forms, Negro Interprofessional Commission on Child Development, (1941-1946).

Division of School Health Services Correspondence and Reports, 1938-1947. Negro Postgraduate Steering Committee, 1940-1941. Post graduate Assembly for Negro Physicians, 1937-1938. Other materials concerning minorities are dispersed throughout the Department of Health records. These materials cannot be identified by title alone.

Rosenberg City Library
2310 Sealy
Galveston, Texas 77550
>Status: permanent
>Update: none
>Dated: 1938-1981
>Volume: unreported

A small collection consisting of a report, article, photographs and oral history, 1938 and 1981.

Clouser, John H. "1938 Annual Negro Health Report of the Volunteer Health League, Galveston, Texas." This crusade was part of a National program during the 1930s.

Clouser, John H. "A Study of Health Among Negroes in Galveston, Texas," 1938.

Oral History of John H. Clouser. Mr. Clouser describes his role as liaison between the African American community and the Caucasian American medical community during the 1930s.

Photographs of Mr. Clouser's public health projects.

University of Texas, Medical Branch
Moody Medical Library.
The blocker history of medicine collections.
>Status: permanent
>Update: periodic
>Dated: 1939-1973
>Volume: 2 documents
>Hours: 8:00 a.m. - 5:00 p.m. Monday-Friday

History of Medicine, 1850-1973. Books (1850-1920), pamphlets (1890-1920) and letters (1939-1973). Collections: F.J.L. Blasingame Papers, (1954-1968), civil rights and minority medical education, and one manuscript.

Galveston County Medical Society Records, 1939-1950. A Society of African American Physicians. Materials include a manuscript.

Hispanics

University of Texas
Health Sciences Center at San Antonio Archives
7703 Floyd Curl Drive
San Antonia, Texas 78284
> Status: permanent
> Update: none
> Dated: 1890-1927
> Volume: unreported

David Cerna Manuscript Collection, Physician, 1890-1927. Writings of a local Hispanic physician include pamphlets (1920-1927) and typescript (1890).

UTAH

No Collection Reported

VERMONT

No Collection Reported

VIRGINIA

Hispanics

University of Virginia
Claude Moore Health Sciences Library
Box 234
Charlottesville, Virginia 22908
> Status: permanent
> Update: none
> Dated: unreported
> Volume: unreported

Walter Reed-Yellow Fever Archive. Contains material mentioning Dr. Reed's work with Cuban volunteers.

WASHINGTON

No Collections Reported

WEST VIRGINIA

African Americans

West Virginia Division of Culture and History
Archives Library Cultural Center - Capitol Complex
1900 Kanawha Boulevard, East
Charleston, West Virginia 25305-0300
> Status: permanent
> Update: none
> Dated: 1909-1957
> Volume: 102 linear feet

State Board of Control Records, 1909-1957. Permanent collection not being updated. 102 linear feet. Material include correspondence and records of segregated hospitals, sanitariums and institutions. These institutions are:
West Virginia School for the Colored Deaf and Blind (Institute, WV)
Denmar Sanitarium (Denmar,WV)
West Virginia Home for the Colored Aged and Infirm (McKendree, WV)
West Virginia Home for the Colored Insane (Lakin, WV)
Contents include: biennial reports (1910- 1951), manuscript boxes of letters (1901-1957), minute books (1917-1957) and correspondence books (1909-1933).

West Virginia Medical Society Records, 1922-1981. Permanent collection not being update. 3000 pieces of material. The West Virginia Medical Society composed of African American Physicians, Dentists and Pharmacists was organized in 1905. Certificate of

Incorporation was received on July 28, 1949. The objects and purposes of the Society shall be to extend medical, dental, and pharmaceutical knowledge and advance to the allied education, to secure the enforcement of just medical laws; to promote friendly intercourse among physicians, dentists, and pharmacists; to guard and foster the material interest to members. Several governor's letters are also contained therein. Correspondence (1932-1979), newspaper clippings, financial materials, printed programs (1938-1953) and reports regarding attendance, care and management of problems found at the W.V. Colored TB Sanitarium and on community non-profit hospitals.

West Virginia State College
Drain-Jordan Library
Institute, West Virginia 25112
      Status: permanent
      Update: none
      Dated: 1940
      Volume: 1 box

Negro Health News, 1940s.

WISCONSIN

No Collections Reported

WYOMING

Native Americans

Wyoming Department of Commerce
Cultural Resoures Division
Barrett Building
Cheyenne, Wyoming 82002-024
      Status: permanent
      Update: none
      Dated: 1887-1995

Volume: unreported

Books and Articles: *"Medicine Among the American Indians*," by Encstone, New York, Hafner Publishing Co., 1962. *"The Medicine Men and Historians of Indian Tribes*," by Jean M. Barrett, WPA subject file 1164. *"The Medicine Men of the Apache*," by John Gregory Bourke, Glorieta, N.M. Rio Grande Press, 1970. *"The Medicine Men of the Apache*," by John C. Bourke, Annual Report of the Bureau of Ethnology, 9th Annual Report, 1887-1888, pp. 443-603. *"Medicine Ceremony of the Menomini, Iowa and Wahpeton Dakota*," by Alanson B. Skinner, New York, Museum of the American Indian, Heve Foundation, 1920. *"Medicine Observations on the Suni Indian*," by Henri Craig, Flemming, New York, Museum of the American Indian, Heve Foundation, 1924. *"Medical Practices and Health in the Choctaw Nation 1831-1885*," by Virginia Rauen, Chronicles of Oklahoma, 48(1):60-73, 1970. "*My Travels with Medicine Man John Lame Peer*," by Richard Erddes, Smithsonian 4(2):30-37, 1973. *The Sham's Healing Way*, by Spencer L. Rogers, Romona, CA, Acona Books, 1976. *"The Story of the White Women Who Lived Among the Arapahoes*," WPA Subject File 707.0.8

BIBLIOGRAPHY

A National Conference on Health Policy, Planning, and Financing the Future of Health Care for Blacks in America. Hyattsville, Maryland: U.S. Department of Health, Education, and Welfare, Public Health Service, National Center for Health Services Research, 1978.

A National Multicultural Seminar on Mental Retardation Among Minority Disadvantaged Populations. Norfolk: Norfolk State College, 1979.

Adams-Esquivel, Henry and Jaime Sena-Rivera (eds.) *The Spanish-Speaking Mental Health Patient.* San Diego: University of California, 1980.

An Assessment of Admission Criteria for Bilingual/BiculturalApplicants to Health Professions Schools. Rockville, Maryland: U.S. Department of Health, Education, and Welfare, Public Health Service, Health Resources Administration, Bureau of Health Manpower, 1979.

An Assessment of Bilingual/Bicultural Awareness Activities in Health Professions Schools. Hyattsville, Maryland: U.S. Department of Health, Education, and Welfare, Public Health Service, Health Resources Administration, 1980.

Arizona Indian Vital Statistics. Tuscon: Indian Health Service, Health Program System Center, Health Status Surveillance Staff, 1967.

Austin, Gregory (ed.) *Drugs and Minorities.* Rockville, Maryland: National Institute on Drug Abuse, 1977.

Asian American Field Survey. Washington: Department of Health, Education, and Welfare, Office of Special Concerns, Division of Asian American Affairs, 1977.

Assessment of Strategies to Promote Cost and Management of Efficiencies in Tribal and Contract Health Service Programs: Final Report. Rockville, MD: Department of Health and Human Services, Public Health Service,Indian Health Service, Office of Planning, Evaluation, and Legislation, Division of Program Evaluation and Policy Analysis, 1990.

Baatz, Wilmer and Phyllis Klotman. *The Black Family and the Black Woman: A Bibliography.* New York: Arno Press, 1978.

Bailey, Eric J. *Urban African American Health Care.* Lanham: University Press of America, c1991.

Bakewell, Dennis. "Science and Medicine." *The Black Experience in the United States.* Northridge, California: n.p., 1970, p. 127.

Barbano, Joseph, Anna Ruth Crocker, and Alice Fusillo. *Minorities and Women in the Health Fields: Applicants, Students, and Workers.* Bethesda, Maryland: U.S. Bureau of Health Resources Development, 1974.

Barbarin, Oscar (ed.) *Institutional Racism and Community Competence.* Rockville, Maryland: U.S. Department of Health and Human Services, Public Health Service, 1982.

Barnes, Nell. *Black Aging: An Annotated Bibliography.* Monticello, Illinois: Vance Bibliographies, 1979.

Barresi, Charles M., Donald E. Stull (eds.). *Ethnic Elderly and Long Term Care.* New York: Springer Publishing Company, c1993.

Barrow, Mark V., Robert Fortuine, Jerry D. Niswander. *Health and Disease of American Indians North of Mexico: A bibliography, 1800-1969.* Gainesville: University of Florida Press, 1972.

Becerra, Rosina M. *Hispanics Seek Health Care: A Study of 1,088 Veterans of Three War Eras.* Lanham, MD, University Press of America, c1983.

Bibliography Committee, New Jersey Library Association, "Social and Economic Conditions." *New Jersey and the Negro: A Bibliography, 1715-1966.* Trenton: The New Jersey Library Association, 1967, pp. 107-116.

Bibliography on Racism, 1972-1975. Rockville, Maryland: U.S. Department of Health, Education, and Welfare, Public Health Service, Alcohol, Drug Abuse, and Mental Health Administration, National Institute of Mental Health, Center for Minority Group Mental Health Program, 1972.

Braithwaite, Ronald L. and Sandra E. Taylor (eds.). *Health Issues in the Black Community.* San Francisco: Jossey-Bass, c1992.

Bureau of Medical Services, Indian Health Service, National Health Service Corps: Grow with Us. Rockville, MD: Department of Health, Education, and Welfare, Public Health Service, Health Services Administration, 1980.

Bush, James A. (ed.) *Suicide and Blacks.* New York: MSS Information Corporation, 1975.

Cabella-Argandona, Roberto, Juan Gomez-Quinones and Patricia Herrera Paran. "Health and Nutrition." *The Chicano: A Comprehensive Bibliographic Study.* Los Angeles, California: Chicano Studies Center, University of California at Los Angeles, 1975, pp. 148-161.

Calling From the Rim: Suicidal Behavior Among American Indian and Alaska Native Adolescents. Denver, CO: The National Center for American Indian and Alaska Native Mental Health Research Center, c 1993.

Cash, Eugene. *Mental Health From A Black Perspective.* Washington: Institute for Urban Affairs and Research, Howard University, 1976.

Cashman, Marc (ed.). "American Indians: Health Care." *Bibliography of American Ethnology.* New York: Todd Publications, 1976, p. 43.

Challenge of the Indian Health Service. Rockville, MD: Department of Health, Education, and Welfare, Public Health Service, Health Services Administration, Bureau of Medical Services, 1979.

Clough, Lynn and T. Neal Garland. *Ethnicity and Health: A Bibliography.* Monticello, Illinois: Vance Bibliographies, 1979.

Cobb, John C. (ed.) *Emotional Problems of Indian Students in Boarding Schools and Related Public Schools.* Albuquerque, N.M.: 1960.

Comparing Serum Ferritin Values from Different Population Surveys. Hyattsville, MD: U.S. Department of Health and Human Services, Public Health Service, Centers for Disease Control, National Center for Health Statistics, 1991.

Conference on Information on Indian Health. Washington: U.S. Department of Health, Education, and Welfare, Public Health Service, 1963.

Cordasco, Francesco. *Useful Spanish for Medical and Hospital Personnel: With a Bibliography on Hispanic Peoples in the United States.* Detroit: Blaine Ethridge Books, 1977.

Data on Earned Degrees Conferred by Institutions of Higher Education by Race, Ethnicity, and Sex, Academic Year 1976- 1977. Washington, D.C.: Department of Health, Education and Welfare, Office for Civil Rights, 1979.

Davis, Cary, Carl Haub and JoAnne Willette. *U.S. Hispanics: Changing the Face of America.* Washington: Population Reference Bureau, 1983.

Davis, Lenwood and Janet Sims. *The Black Family in the United States.* Westport, Connecticut: Greenwood Press, 1978.

Davis, Lenwood G. *A History of Public Health, Health Problems, Facilities, and Services in the Black Community.* Monticello, Illinois: council of Planning Librarians, 1975.

Davis, Lenwood G. *A History of Tuberculosis in the Black Community: A Working Bibliography.* Monticello, Illinois: Council of Planning Librarians, 1975.

Davis, Lenwood G. *The History of Selected Diseases in the Black Community: A Working Bibliography.* Monticello, Illinois: Council of Planning Librarians, 1976.

Davis, Lenwood G. *The Mental Health of the Black Community: An Exploratory Bibliography.* Monticello, Illinois: council of Planning Librarians, 1975.

Davis, Lenwood. *The Black Aged in the United States: An Annotated Bibliography.* Westport, Connecticut: Greenwood Press, 1980.

Davis, Morris and Andrew Rowland. *The Occupational Health of Black Workers: A Bibliography.* Monticello, Illinois: Vance Bibliographies, 1980.

Dawson, Deborah. *Aids Knowledge and Attitudes of Black Americans: Provisional Data from the 1988 National Health Interview Survey.* Hyattsville, MD: U.S. Department of Health and Human Services, Public Health Service, Centers for Disease Control, 1989.

Dennis, C.A.R. and B.L. Pearson. *The Effects of the Living Environment on the Health of Saskatchewan Indians.* Regina: Prarie Institute of Environmental Health, 1978.

Dental Services for American Indians and Alaska Natives. Rockville, Maryland: U.S. Department of Health, Education, and Welfare, Public Health Service, etc., 1964-65.

Dental Services for Indians. Washington: U.S. Dept. of Health, Education, and Welfare, Public Health Service, Bureau of Medical Services, Division of Indian Health, 1958-1961.

Dental Services for Indians. Washington: U.S. Dept. of Health, Education, and Welfare, Public Health Service, Bureau of Medical Services, Division of Indian Health, 1964.

Disease Patterns: Black Health Status in Georgia. Atlanta, Georgia: Georgia Department of Human Resources, Division of Physical Health, Health Services Research and Statistics Section, 1975.

Dixon, Barbara M. *Good Health for African Americans.* New York: Crown, c1994.

Doi, Mary L. *Pacific Asian American Research; An Annotated Bibliography.* Chicago, IL, Pacific Asian American Mental Health Research Center, c1981.

Dula, Annette and Sara Goering (eds.). *"It Just Ain't Fair": The Ethics of Health Care for African Americans.* Westport, CT: Praeger, 1994.

Eligibility for Health Care Services Provided by Indian Health Service. Washington: United States Congress, Sentate, and Select Committee on Indian Affairs, 1988.

Findings from the Survey of American Inidians and Alaska Natives Health Care Coverage. Rockville, MD: Agency for Health Care Policy and Research, 1992.

Findings from the Survey of American Indians and Alaska Natives Access to Health Care. Rockville, MD: Agency for Health Care Policy and Research, 1992.

First Conference on Hypertension Among Puerto Ricans. Bethesda, Maryland: U.S. Department of Health, Education, and Welfare, Public Health Service, National Institutes of Health, 1980.

Frank-Stromborg, Marilyn and Sharon J. Olsen (eds.). *Cancer Prevention in Minority Populations: Cultural Implications for Health Care Professionals.* St. Louis, Mosby, c1993.

Fortuine, Robert. *The Health of the Eskimos; A Bibliography, 1857-1967.* Hangover, New Hampshire: Dartmouth College Libraries, 1968.

Furino, Antonio (ed.) *Health Policy and the Hispanic.* Boulder: Westview Press, 1992.

Garcia-Avenues, Franciso, Darien Fisher, and Hilda Villarreal. "Health." *Quicu Sabe? A Preliminary List of Chicano Reference Materials.* Los Angeles: Chicano Studies Research Center Publication, 1981, pp. 86-89.

Garcia-Avenues, Franciso, Darien Fisher, and Hilda Villasreal. "Medicine." *Quicu Sabe? A Preliminary List of Chicano Reference Materials.* Los Angeles, California: Bibliographic and Reference Series No. 11, Chicago Studies Research Center Publication, University of California at Los Angeles, 1981, p. 53.

Ginzberg, Eli. *Medical Gridlock and Health Reform.* Boulder, CO: Westview Press, 1994.

Guide to the Utilization of Family and Community Support Systems by Pacific Asian Elderly. Washington, D.C.: National Pacific Asian Resource Center on Aging, 1985.

Habermacher, Joan. *Hispanic Health Services Research.* Hyattsville, Maryland: U.S. Department of Health and Human Services, Public Health Service, Office of Health Research, Statistics, and Technology, National Center for Health Services Research, 1980.

Hanson, Roger K. "Health and Medicine." *Black Bibliography: University of Utah Marriott Library.* Salt Lake City, Utah: University of Utah, Marriott Library, pp. 368-372.

Harper, Frederick (ed.) *Alcoholism Treatment and Black Americans.* Rockville, Maryland; U.S. Department of Health, Education and Welfare, Public Health Service, Alcohol, Drug Abuse and Mental Health Administration, National Institute on Alcohol Abuse and Alcoholism, Division of Special Treatment and Rehabilitation, 1979.

Hausner, Tony. *Health of the Disadvantaged Chart Book.* Hyattsville, Maryland: U.S. Department of Health, Education, and Welfare, Public Health Service, Health Resources Administration, Office of Health Resources Opportunity, 1977.

Health and Nutrition: Collection of Vital Statistical Data on Hispanics: Briefing Report to Congressional Requesters. Washington, D.C.: General Accounting Office, 1988.

Health Careers for American Indians and Alaska Natives: A Source Book. Washington, D.C., 1970.

Health Indicators for Hispanic, Black and White Americans. Hyattsville, MD: U.S. Department of Health and Human Services, Public Health Service, National Center for Health Statistics, 1984.

Health of Black and White Americans, 1985-87. Hyattsville, MD: U.S. Department of Health and Human Services, Public Health Service, Centers for Disease Control, National Center for Health Statistics, 1990.

Health Services Administration: Bureau of Community Health Services, Indian Health Service, Bureau of Medical Services.. Rockville, MD: Departmen tof Health, Education, and Welfare, Public Health Service, Health Services Administration, 1979.

Heart Disease Among Indians. Washington, 1957. Howe, Mentor A. and Rosecoe H. Lewis. "Negro Health, Housing and Social Conditions." *A Classified Catalogue of the Negro Collection in the Collis P. Huntington Library, Hampton Institute.* Detroit: Negro History Press, 1940, 1971, pp. 227-230.

Hultkrantz, Ake. *Shamanic Healing and Ritual Drama: Health and Medicine in Native North American Religious Traditions.* New York: Crossroad, 1992.

Iiyama, Patti, Setsuko Matsunaga Nishi, Bruce D. Johnson. *Drug Use and Abuse Among U.S. Minorities.* New York: Praeger, 1976.

Indian Health Highlights. Washington: U.S. Department of Health, Education, and Welfare, Public Health Service, Bureau of Medical Services, Division of Indian Health, Office of Program Planning and Evaluation, Program Analysis and Statistics Branch, 1956-1966.

Indian Health Program, 1955-1980. Rockville, MD: Department of Health and Human Services, Public Health Service, Health Services Administration, 1980.

Indian Health Program of the United States Public Health Service. Rockville, MD: Department of Health, Education and Welfare, Public Health Service, Health Services Administration, Indian Health Services.

Indian Health Service. Washington, D.C.: U.S. Department of Health and Human Resources, Public Health Service, Health Resources and Services Administration, 1985.

Indian Health Service: A Comprehensive Health Care Program for American Indians and Alaska Natives. Rockville, MD: U.S. Department of Health and Human Services, Public Health Service, Health Resources and Services Administration, Indian Health Service, 1985.

Indian Health Service "Chart Series" Tables. Rockville, Maryland: Office of Program Statistics, Division of Resource Coordination, Indian Health Service, 1982.

Indian Health Service Clinician's Guide to Resources. Phoenix, AZ: The Clinical Support Center, 1985.

Indian Vital Statistics, Oklahoma Area. Tucson: Indian Health Service, Health Program Systems Center, Health Status Surveillance Staff, 1967-68.

Indian Vital Statistics, Portland Area. Tucson: Indian Health Service, Health Program System Center, Health Status Surveillance Staff, 1968.

Indian Vital Statistics, South Dakota. Tucson: Health Program Systems Center, Indian Health Service, 1967.

Indian Vital Statistics. Tucson: Indian Health Service, Health Program Systems Center, Health Status Surveillance Staff, 1968.

Indian Vital Statistics. Tucson: Office of Program Development, Indian Health Service, 1969.

Information on Indian Health. Washington: U.S. Dept. of Health, Education, and Welfare, Public Health Service, 1963.

Irish, Donald P., Kathleen F. Lindquist, Vivian Jenkins Nelsen (eds.). *Ethnic Variations in Dying, Death, and Grief: Diversity in Universality.* Washington, D.C.: Taylor & Francis, c1993.

Johnson, Ernest H. *Risky Sexual Behaviors Among African-Americans.*
    Westport, CT: Praeger, 1993.

Jones, Woodrow, Jr. and Mitchell F. Rice (eds.) *Health Care Issues in Black
    America: Policies, Problems, and Prospects.* New York: Green-
    wood Press, 1987.

Jordan, Lois. "Health and Psychology." *Mexican Americans: Resources to
    Build Cultural Understanding.* Littleton, Colorado: Libraries
    Unlimited, 1973, pp. 68-71.

Jordan, Lois. "Health and Psychology." *Mexican Americans: Resources to
    Build Cultural Understanding.* Littleton, Colorado: Libraries
    Unlimited, Inc., 1973, pp. 68-71.

Justice, James. *Bibliography of Health and Disease in North American
    Indians, Eskimos and Aluets, 1969 to 1979.* Tucson: U.S. Depart-
    ment of Health and Human Services, Public Health Service, Health
    Resources and Service Administration, Indian Health Service, Office
    of Research and Development, 1982.

Kansas Indian Vital Statistics. Tucson: Division of Indian Health, Health
    Program Systems Center, Health Status Surveillance Staff, 1967.

Keehn, Pauline. *The Effect of Epidemic Diseases on the Natives of North
    America: An Annotated Bibliography.* London: Survival Interna-
    tional, 1978.

Kelso, Dianne and Carolyn Attneave. *Bibliography of North American
    Indian Mental Health.* Westport, Connecticut: Greenwood Press,
    1981.

Kenton, Charlotte. *Health Needs and Services for Hispanic Americans:
    January 1980 Through July 1982.* Bethesda, Maryland: U.S.
    Department of Health and Human Services, Public Health Service,
    National Institutes of Health, 1982.

Kirkwood, Kenneth (ed.) *Biosocial Aspects of Ethnic Minorities.*
    Cambridge, England: Galton Foundation, 1983.

Klein, Barry T. *Reference Encyclopedia of the American Indian.* Rye, New York: Todd Publications, 1973-1974.

Koba Associates. *The Treatment Practices of Black Physicians.* Rockville, Maryland: U.S. Department of Health, Education, and Welfare, Public Health Service, Health Resources Administration, 1979.

Kunitz, Stephen J. *Navajo Aging: The Transition From Family to Institutional Support.* Tucson: University of Arizona Press, c1991.

LeRiche, W. Harding. *A Health Survey of African Children in Alexandra Township.* Johannesburg: Witwatersand University Press, 1943.

Loytued, Dagmar. "Psychology and Health." *Afro-American Studies, Volume 2.* Berlin, Germany: John F. Kennedy Institute Library, 1981, pp.473-475.

Lucas, Vivian. *Health of the Disadvantaged Chart Book-II.* Hyattsville, Maryland: U.S. Department of Health and Human Services, Public Health Service, Health Resources Administration, Office of Health Resources Opportunity, 1980.

Luckraft, Dorothy (ed.) *Black Awareness: Implications for Black Patient Care.* New York: American Journal of Nursing Company, 1976.

Lyon, Juana (ed.) *The Indian Elder, A Forgotten American.* Washington, D.C.: National Tribal Chairman's Association, 1978.

Malzberg, Benjamin. *Statistical Data for the Study of Mental Disease Among Negroes in New York State, 1939–1941.* Albany, 1955.

Malzberg, Benjamin. *Statistical Data for the Study of Mental Disease Among Negroes in New York State, 1949–1951.* Albany, 1959.

Malzberg, Benjamin. *The Mental Health of the Negro.* Albany: Research Foundation for Mental Hygiene, 1962-1963.

Martinez, Joe. *Chicano Psychology.* New York: Academic Press, 1977.

McIntosh, John. *Suicide Among U.S. Racial Minorities: A Comprehensive Bibliography.* Monticello, Illinois: Vance Bibliographies, 1981.

Melnick, Vijaya and Franklin Hamilton (eds.) *Minorities in Science: The Challenge for Change in Biomedicine.* New York: Plenum Press, 1977.

Miller, Elizabeth W., and Mary L. Fisher. "Health." *The Negro in America: A Bibliography.* Cambridge, Massachusetts: Harvard University Press, 1970, pp. 59-68.

Miller, Elizabeth. "Health." *The Negro in America: A Bibliography.* Cambridge, Massachusetts: Harvard University Press, 1966, pp. 33-39.

Miller, Helen and Ernest Mason (eds.) *Contemporary Minority Leaders in Nursing: Afro-American, Hispanic, and American Perspectives.* Kansas City, Missouri: American Nurses Association, 1983.

Minnesota Indian People: Selected Health Statistics. Minneapolis: 1980.

Minority Biomedical Support Program. Bethesda, Maryland: U.S. Department of Health and Human Services, Public Health Service, National Institutes of Health, 1980.

Minority Groups in Medicine: Selected Bibliography. Bethesda, Maryland: U.S. Government Printing Office, 1972.

Minority Groups in Nursing 1976: A Bibliography. Kansas City, Missouri: American Nurses' Association, 1976.

Minority Groups in Nursing: A Selected Bibliography. Kansas City, Missouri: American Nurses' Association, 1973.

Minority Student Opportunities in United States Medical Schools. Washington, D.C.: Association of American Medical College, 1969/70.

Miralles, Maria Andrea. *A Matter of Life and Death: Health-Seeking Behavior of Guatemalan Refugees in South Florida.* New York: AMS Press, c1989.

Mississippi Indian Vital Statistics. Tucson: Division of Indian Health, Health Program Systems Center, Health Status Surveillance Staff, 1967.

Mitchell, Parren J. *"Affirmative Action: Social Security can do more to improve African Americans representation in its work force."* Washington: U.S. General Accounting Office, 1987.

Momeni, Jamohid A. "Black Health and Mortality." *Demography of the Black Population in the United States.* Westport, Connecticut: Greenwood Press, 1983, pp. 203-234.

Moore, Thomas, Amelie Gutierrez Ramirez, and Patricia Slayton (eds.) *Proceedings of the Conference on Communicating with Mexican Americans on Their Good Health.* Bethesda, Maryland: U.S. Department of Health and Human Service, Public Health Service, National Institutes of Health, 1982.

Moore, William M., Marjorie M. Silverberg and Merrill S. Read (eds.) *Nutrition, Growth, and Development of North American Indian Children.* Washington, U.S. Government Printing Office, 1972.

Murata, Alice K. and Judith Farquhar (eds.) *Issues in Pacific_Asian American Health and Mental Health: A Report of a P/AAMHRC Task Force.* Chicago, IL, Pacific Asian American Mental Health Research Center, c1982.

Murdock, George Peter. *Ethnographic Bibliography of North America.* New Haven: Human Relations Area Files, 1960.

Murguia, Edward. *Ethnicity and Aging, a Bibliography.* San Antonio: Trinity University Press, 1984.

Myers, Hectors, Phyllis G. Rana and Marcia Harris. "Physical Development." *Black Child Development in America, 1927-1977.* Westport, Connecticut: Greenwood Press, 1979, pp. 45-84.

Myers, Hector, Phyllis Rana, and Marcia Harris. *Black Child Development in America, 1927-1977: An Annotated Bibliography.* Westport, Connecticut: Greenwood Press, 1979.

Nandi, Proshanta K. *The Quality of Life of Asian Americans: An Exploratory Study in a Middle-Size Community.* Chicago, IL: Pacific Asian American Mental Health Research Center, c1980.

National Concern: Diabetes in Black Americans. Bethesda, MD: U.S. Department of Health and Human Services, Public Health Service, National Institutes of Health, National Institute of Diabetes, Digestive, and Kidney Diseases, 1991.

National Conference on Asian-American Mental Health. Rockville, Maryland: National Institute of Mental Health, Center for Minority Group Mental Health Programs, 1972.

National Health Care Reform and Its Implications for Indian Health Care. Washington: United States Congress, Senate, Committee on Indian Affairs, 1994.

Newman, Richard. *Black Access: A Bibliography of Afro-American Bibliographies.* Westport, Connecticut: Greenwood Press, 1984.

Newton, Frank, Esteban Olmedo, Amado Padilla. *Hispanic Mental Health Research.* Berkeley: University of California Press, 1982.

North Dakota Indian Vital Statistics. Tucson: Indian Health Service, Health Program Systems Center, Health Status Surveillance Staff, 1967.

Opportunities in Nursing. Aberdeen, South Dakota: Indian Health Service - Aberdeen Area, 1980.

Oral Health Program, Division of Indian Health; Annual Report. Washington: U.S. Department of Health, Education, and Welfare, Public Health Service, Division of Indian Health, Dental Services Branch, 1958.

Padilla, Amado and Eligio Padilla (eds.) *Improving Mental Health and Human Services for Hispanic Communities.* Washington: National Coalition of Hispanic Mental Health and Human Service Organizations, 1977.

Padilla, Amado M. and Paul Aranda. *Latino Mental Health*. Rockville, Maryland: Alcohol, Drug Abuse, and Mental Health Administration, 1974.

Pathways to a Career in Dentistry: A Sourcebook for Students Under-Represented in Dentistry. Cambridge, Massachusetts: Tufts University, School of Dental Medicine, 1974.

Pino, Frank. "Medicine and Health." *Mexican Americans: A Research Bibliography, Volume 2*. East Lansing: Michigan State University, 1974, pp. 278-292.

Porter, Dorothy R. "Medicine and Health." *The Negro in the United States: A Selected Bibliography*. Washington, D.C.: Library of Congress, 1970, pp. 195-199.

Porter, Dorothy. "Medicine and Health." *A Working Bibliography on the Negro in the United States*. Ann Arbor, Michigan: University Microfilms, 1969, pp. 172-176.

Powell, Mary Lucas, Patricia S. Bridges, Ann Marie Wagner Mires (eds.) *What Mean These Bones?: Studies in Southeastern Bioarchaeology*. Tuscaloosa: University of Alabama Press, c1991.

Prevalence of Know Diabetes Among Black Americans. Hyattsville, MD: U.S. Department of Health and Human Services, Public Health Service, National Center for Health Statistics, 1987.

Proceedings of the Second Minority Hypertension Research Development Summer Program Seminar. Bethesda, Maryland: U.S. Department of Health, Education, and Welfare, Public Health Service, National Institutes of Health, 1979.

Proceedings on the 1980 Forum on Hypertension in Minority Populations. Bethesda, Maryland: U.S. Department of Health and Human Services, Public Health Service, National Institutes of Health, 1982.

Puerto Ricans in Science and Biomedicine: Report of a Conference. Washington, D.C.: American Association for the Advance of Science, 1981.

R.J. Associates. *Asian American Reference Data Directory.* Washington, Office for Asian American Affairs, 1976.

Reed, Katherine. *Mental Health and Social Services for Mexican-Americans: An Essay and Annotated Bibliography.* Monticello, Illinois: Council of Planning Librarians, 1976.

Reed, Wornie L. *Health and Medical Care of African-Americans.* Westport, CT: Auburn House, 1993.

Rice, Mitchell F. *Health of Black Americans From Post Reconstruction to Integration, 1871–1860: An Annotated Bibliography of Contemporary Sources.* Connecticut: Greenwood Press, 1990.

Riley, Susan G. (ed.) *Proceedings, Mental Health Planning Conference for the Spanish Speaking.* Rockville, Maryland: National Institute of Mental Health, 1972.

Robinson, Barbara, J. Cordell Robinson, and Carlos E. Cartes. "Social and Behavioral Sciences." *The Mexican American: A Critical Guide to Research Aids.* Greenwich, Connecticut: JAI Press, Inc, 1980, pp. 203-224.

Rogler, Lloyd H. *Hispanics and Mental Health: A Framework for Research.* Malabar, FL, R.E. Krieger Publishing Company, 1989.

Rosenstein, Marilyn. *Hispanic Americans and Mental Health Services.* Rockville, Maryland: U.S. Department of Health and Human Services, Public Health Service, Alcohol, Drug Abuse, and Mental Health Administration, National Institute of Mental Health Administration, 1980.

Sanders, Charles (ed.) *Mental Health Programs for Racial Minorities.* Washington: Mental Health Research and Development Center, Institute for Urban Affairs and Research, Howard University, 1977.

Sanjur, Diva. *Hispanic Foodways, Nutrition, and Health.* Boston, Allyn and Bacon, c1995.

Sammons, Vivian O and Denise P Dempsey. "Blacks in Science and Related Disciplines. Washington: Library of Congress, 1989.

Sata, Lindberg and Keh-Ming Lin (eds.) *Culturally Relevant Training for Asian American Psychiatrists.* Washington: American Psychiatric Association, 1977.

Schatz, Walter. *Directory of Afro-American Resources.* New York: R.R. Bowker Company, 1970.

Second Annual Rocky Mountain Mental Health Conference on Minority Groups. Boulder, Colorado: Western Center for Continuing Education in Mental Health, Western Interstate Commission for Higher Education, 1979.

Selected Bibliography on Ethnic and Racial Factors in Hypertension. Bethesda, Maryland: National Institutes of Health, 1980.

Serafica, Felicisima C. (ed). *Mental Health of Ethnic Minorities*, New York, Praeger, 1990.

Sharpley, Robert. *Treatment Issues: Foreign Medical Graduates and Black Patient Populations.* Cambridge, Massachusetts: Solomon Fuller Institute, 1977.

Silverberg, Edwin and Cyril Poindexter. *Cancer Facts and Figures for Black Americans, 1979.* New York: American Cancer Society, 1979.

Simmons, Jeannette (ed.) *Making Health Education Work: Health Education in Health Program Development, with Primary Attention on Programming for Low-Income and Minority Groups.* Washington: American Public Health Association, 1976.

Sims, Janet L. and Bettye Thomas. "Health and Beauty." *The Progress of Afro-American Women.* Westport, Connecticut: Greenwood Press, 1980, pp. 163-167.

Sims, Janet L. and Bettye Thomas. "Medicine, Nursing and Related Areas." *The Progress of Afro-American Women.* Westport, Connecticut: Greenwood Press, 1980, pp. 215-235.

Smith, Benjamin. *Afro-American History: A Bibliography.* Santa Barbara, California: ABC-CLIO, Inc., 1974.

Smith, Dwight. "The Contemporary Scene (Since 1945)." *Afro-American History, Volume II*. Santa Barbara, California: ABC-CLIO Press, 1981, pp. 173-259.

Smith, Melody A. *Minorities and the Health Professions: An Annotated Bibliography*. Washington: Division of Student Affairs, Association of American Medical Colleges, 1972.

Sotomayor, Marta (ed.) *Empowering Hispanic Families: A Critical Issue for the '90s*. Milwaukee, WS: Family Service America, c1991.

Souflee, Federico Jr. and George Valdez (eds.) *Proceedings of the Texas-New Mexico Symposium on the Delivery of Mental Health Services to Mexican Americans*. Houston: Chicano Training Center, 1978.

Southeast Asian American Food Habits. Washington: Department of Agriculture, Food and Nutrition Service.

Spradling, Mary Mace (ed.) *In Black and White: A Guide to Magazine Articles, Newspaper Articles, and Books Concerning More than 15,000 Black Individuals and Groups*. Detroit: Gale Research Company, 1980.

Stanford, E. Percil (ed.) *Comprehensive Service Delivery Systems for the Minority Aged*. San Diego: Center on Aging, School of Social Work, San Diego State University, 1978.

Stanford, E. Percil (ed.) *Minority Aging Research : Old Issues-New Approaches*. San Diego: University Center on Aging, College of Human Services, San Diego State University, 1979.

Stanford, E. Percil (ed.) *Minority Aging*. San Diego, California: Center on Aging, School of Social Work, San Diego State University, 1974.

Stanford, E. Percil (ed.) *Minority Aging: Policy Issues for the '80s*. San Diego: University Center on Aging, College of Human Services, San Diego State University, 1981.

Stanford, E. Percil (ed.) *Retirement, Concepts and Realities of Ethnic Minority Elders*. San Diego: University Center on Aging, College of Human Services, San Diego State University, 1978.

Status of Dental Health in the Black Community: Final Report. Baltimore: 1973.

Street, Pamela, Ronald Wood and Riga Chowenhill. *Alcohol Use Among Native Americans.* Berkeley: Social Research Group, School of Public Health, University of California, 1976.

Sturtevant, William C. *Bibliography on American Indian Medicine and Health.* Washington: Smithsonian Institute, 1962.

Sue, Stanley and James K. Morishima. *The Mental Health of Asian Americans.* San Francisco: Jossey-Bass, 1982.

Suicide Among the American Indians. Chevy Chase, Maryland: National Institute of Mental Health, 1969.

Summary Report of the National Indian Conference on Aging. Phoenix, Arizona: The Conference, 1976.

Summary Report on the National Symposium on High Blood Pressure Control in U.S. Asian and Pacific Populations. Bethesda, Maryland: U.S. Department of Health, Education and Welfare, Public Health Service, National Institutes of Health, 1978.

Talbot, Jane and Gilbert R. Cruz. "Health: Physical and Mental." *A Comprehensive Chicano Bibliography, 1960-1972.* Austin: Jenkins Publishing Company, 1973, pp. 210-223.

Teicher, Morton I. *Windigo Psychosis: A Study of a Relationship Between Belief and Behavior Among the Indians of Northeastern Canada.* Seattle: American Ethnological Society, 1960.

The Health Team and the Health Care of the Urban Black. 1977.

The Minority Elderly in America, an Annotated Bibliography. Washington, D.C.: Department of Health, Education, and Welfare, Office of Human Development Services, Administration on Aging, 1980.

Thompson, Edgart and Alma M. Thompson. "The American Negro Population." *Race and Region.* Chapel Hill, North Carolina: University of North Carolina Press, 1949, pp. 42-43.

Thompson, Edgart and Alma M. Thompson. "The Negro Physical Type." *Race and Region.* Chapel Hill, North Carolina: University of North Carolina Press, 1949, pp. 48-49.

Thompson, Edgart and Alma M. Thompson. "The Racial Balance of Births and Deaths." *Race and Region.* Chapel Hill, North Carolina: University of North Carolina Press, 1949, pp. 44-47.

Thompson, Edgart and Alma M. Thompson. "White and Negro Intelligence." *Race and Region.* Chapel Hill, North Carolina: University Of North Carolina Press, 1949, pp. 49-53.

Thompson, Theodis and Florence Johnson Hicks (eds.) *Health Policy and Planning in the Urban Community.* Silver Spring, Maryland: Ebon Research Systems, 1975.

Thorne, Kathleen, et al. "Mexican-Americans Health." *Minorities in America.* San Jose, California: San Jose State College Library, 1969, p. 126.

Torrey, E. Fuller. *Community Health and Mental Health Care Delivery for North American Indians.* New York: MSS Information Corp., 1974.

Toward Quality Nursing Care for a Multiracial Society: Toward Quality Nursing Care for a Multiracial Society. Kansas City, Missouri: Affirmative Action Task Force, American Nurses' Association, 1976.

Treiman, Beatrice et al. *Alcohol Use Among the Spanish-Speaking: A Selective Annotated Bibliography.* Berkeley, California: Social Research Group, School of Public Health, University of California, 1976.

Treiman, Beatrice R., Pamela B. Street and Patricia Shanks. *Blacks and Alcohol: A Selective Annotated Bibliography.* Berkeley, California: Social Research Group, School of Public Health, University of California, 1976.

Utah Indian Vital Statistics. Tucson: Indian Health Service, Health Program Systems Center, Health Status Surveillance Staff, 1967.

Velimirovic, Boris (ed.) *Modern Medicine and Medical Anthropology in the United States-Mexico Border Population.*

Washington: Pan American Health Organization, Pan American Sanitary Bureau, Regional Office of the World Health Organization, 1978.

Vohra-Sahu, Indu. *The Pacific Asian Americans: A Selected and Annotated Bibliography of Recent Materials.* Chicago, Illinois: Pacific Asian American Mental Health Research Center, 1983.

Walters, Mary D. "Medicine." *Afro-Americana: A Comprehensive Bibliography of Resource Materials in the Ohio State University Libraries By or About Black Americans.* Columbus, Ohio: Office of Educational Services, The Ohio State University Libraries, 1969, p. 163.

Watson, Wilbur and Brenda Allen (eds.) *Health and the Black Aged.* Washington: Nation Center on Black Aged, 1978.

Waxman, Julia. "Housing, Health and Recreation." *Race Relations.* Chicago: Julius Rosen Wald Fund, 1945, pp. 30-31.

Whitney, Philip B. *America's Third World.* Berkeley: General Library, University of California, 1970.

Williams, Blanch Spruiel. *Characteristics of the Black Elderly.* Washington, D.C.: U.S. Department of Health and Human Services, Office of Human Development Services, Administration on Aging, National Clearinghouse on Aging, 1980.

Wong, Paul. *Minority Community Mental Health Training: Analysis of an Educational Experiment.* Chicago, Ill: Pacific Asian Mental Health Reserach Center, c1986.

Work, Monroe N. "Health Problems of Negroes." *A Bibliography of the Negro in Africa and America.* New York: The H. W. Wilson Company, 1928, pp. 508–527.

Workship on Alternative Indian Health Delivery Systrems, Rockville, MD, March 11-12, 1987: Summary Report. Rockville, MD: U.S.

Department of Health and Human Services, Public Health Service, Health Resources and Services Administration, 1987.

Zuniga, Alfredo. "Superstition, Medicine and Folklore." *Mexico and the Southwest Collection*. Fullerton: California State University, 1977, pp. 215-219.

APPENDIX A:
DATA COLLECTION
QUESTIONNAIRES

HEALTH COLLECTIONS ON ETHNIC
MINORITY POPULATIONS
(Duplicate as Necessary)

Repository Name:————————————————————————

Repository Address:————————————————————————

————————————————————————

Telephone Number:————————————————————————

1.　Is the collection open for public use?————————————————————

　　Time(s) collection open:————————————————————

2.　Contents:

　　a.　Title of collection:————————————————————

　　b.　Please describe your ethnic health collection:

　　　　i.　The origin (inlcude the date this collection began at your institution; the original source of the material; and other pertinent information on how and when the collection was started).

　　　　ii.　Approximate total pieces of material:————————————————

　　　　iii.　Approximate dates of material:
　　　　　　Oldest date ——————— Latest date ———————

　　　　iv.　Is this a permanent or rotating collection? ———————

　　c.　Is the collection being updated? ————————————————

　　　　If yes, how often? ————————————————

d.   List the types of material included in the collection: (Please check the appropriate boxes)

	Approximate Number	Inclusion Dates
☐ Books	_____	_____
☐ Pamphlets	_____	_____
☐ Letters	_____	_____
☐ Articles	_____	_____
☐ Video Tapes	_____	_____
☐ Cassette Tapes	_____	_____
☐ Handbills	_____	_____
☐ Newspaper Clippings	_____	_____
☐ Other _____ Please specify	_____	_____
☐ Other _____ Please specify	_____	_____
☐ Other _____ Please specify	_____	_____

e.   Describe the health area or activity of individual, families, organization or institutions listed in the collection. Please include date of birth and date of death of the individual or formation date of the organization stated in the collection name.

(Please attach additional sheets if necessary)

	• Collection Name • Date of Birth/Death • Date of Collection • Identity of Ethnic Group	Health area(s) or activity area (Pediatrics, Civil Rights, etc.)	Form of material (Book, Articles, etc.)
1			
2			
3			
4			
5			
6			
7			
8			
9			
10			

f. Are there other special characteristics about your collection you wish to discuss? Please state these special features in the space below.

g. Do you have knowledge of other historical collections referencing contributions to the health sciences by ethnic minority populations?

ETHNIC HEALTH COLLECTION
(Duplicate as Necessary)

Contact Person:_____

Title/Position:_____

Address:_____

_____

Telephone Number:_____

1. Are books/pamphlets free to the public? □ Yes   □ No
    A.   If yes, give the address to request the material:
    _____

    _____

    _____

    _____

    B.   If yes, what is the limit on the number of copies? _____ (99= unlimited)

    C.   If no, (books/pamphlets are <u>not free</u>), how can the material be obtained?
    _____

    _____

    _____

    _____

2. Is there a listing of the material currently available? □ yes □ no
    If yes, please send a copy with your completed questionnaire.

3. Is the listing available from the address given in #1-A above? □   yes   □ no
    If no, give the appropriate address:
    _____

    _____

    _____

    _____

4.   Describe material related to ethnic health:

   A.   Approximate dates _____ to _____ .
                              (oldest)   (latest)

   B.   Number of pamphlets_____ .

   C.   Number of books_____ .

   D.   Other (please describe)_____

   _____

5.   Is there a listing of outdated health materials related to ethnic minorities which are not stored
     in your information office but which relate to your agency activities? (For example, to find
     conference proceedings from the 1960's where would the listing be located?)

   _____

   _____

   _____

6.   What are your hours of operation when the public can access your information materials?
     _____ to _____ (times)

     _____ to _____ (days of the week)

7.   Is an appointment necessary to view the holdings? ☐ yes   ☐ no

8.   Do you have a mailing list for materials routinely distributed? ☐ yes   ☐ no

9.   How often are books/pamphlets updated? _____

   _____

APPENDIX B:
LISTING OF LIBRARIES
CONTACTED

Medical Schools

1. Albany Medical College of Union College
    Albany, New York   12208
2. Baylor College of Medicine
    Houston, Texas   77030
3. Boston University School of Medicine
    Boston, Massachusetts 02118
4. Brown University
    Division of Biology and Medicine
    Providence, Rhode Island 02912
5. Case Western Reserve University
    School of Medicine
    Cleveland, Ohio   44106
6. City University of New York
    Mount Sinai School of Medicine
    New York, New York   10029
7. College of Medicine and Dentistry of New Jersey
    New Jersey Medical School
    Newark, New Jersey   07103
8. College of Medicine and Dentistry of New Jersey
    Rutgers Medical School
    Piscataway, New Jersey   08854
9. Columbia University Faculty of Medicine
    New York, New York   10021
10. Cornell University Medical College

New York, New York   10021
11.   Craighton University School of Medicine
      Omaha, Nebraska 68178
12.   Dartmouth Medical School
      Hanover, New Hampshire   03755
13.   Duke University School of Medicine
      Durham, North Carolina 27710
14.   Eastern Virginia Medical School
      School of Medicine
      Norfolk, Virginia 23501
15.   Emory University School of Medicine
      Atlanta, Georgia 30322
16.   Georgetown University School of Medicine
      Washington, D.C.   20007
17.   George Washington University School of Medicine
      Washington, D.C.   20005
18.   Hahnemann Medical College
      Philadelphia, Pennsylvania   19102
19.   Harvard Medical School
      Boston, Massachusetts   02115
20.   Howard University College of Medicine
      Washington, D.C.   20059
21.   Indian University School of Medicine
      Indianapolis, Indiana 46202
22.   Thomas Jefferson University
      Jefferson Medical College
      Philadelphia, Pennsylvania   19107
23.   Johns Hopkins University School of Medicine
      Baltimore, Maryland   21205
24.   Laval University Faculty of Medicine
      Quebec, Que Glk 7P4, Canada
25.   Loma Linda University School of Medicine
      Loma Linda, California 92354
26.   Louisiana State University Medical Center, New Orleans
      New Orleans, Louisiana   70112
27.   Louisiana State University Medical Center
      Shreveport School of Medicine
      Shreveport, Louisiana 71101
28.   Loyola University Stritch School of Medicine
      Maywood, Illinois 60153
29.   McMaster University Division of Health Sciences

Hamilton, Ontario LBS 4L8, Canada
30. Medical College of Georgia
    Augusta, Georgia 30912
31. Medical College of Ohio
    Toledo, Ohio 43614
32. Medical College of Pennsylvania
    Philadelphia, Pennsylvania 19129
33. Medical College of Wisconsin
    Milwaukee, Wisconsin 53226
34. Medical University of South Carolina
    Charleston, South Carolina 29403
35. Meharry Medical College
    Department of Medicine
    Nashville, Tennessee 37208
36. Mercer University Medical School
    Atlanta, Georgia 30341
37. Michigan State University
    College of Human Medicine
    East Lansing, Michigan 48823
38. New York Medical College
    Valhalla, New York 10595
39. New York University School of Medicine
    New York, New York 10016
40. Northwestern University Medical School
    Chicago, Illinois 60611
41. Ohio State University College of Medicine
    Columbus, Ohio 43210
42. Pennsylvania State University Medical Center
    Hershey, Pennsylvania 17033
43. Rush University
    College of Medicine
    Chicago, Illinois 60612
44. Saint Louis University School of Medicine
    St. Louis, Missouri 63104
45. Southern Illinois University School of Medicine
    Springfield, Illinois 62702
46. Stanford University School of Medicine
    Stanford, California 94305
47. State University of New York at Buffalo
    Medical School
    Buffalo, New York 14214

48.   State University of New York at
       Stony Brook Health Sciences Center
       School of Medicine
       Stony Brook, New York   11794

49.   State University of New York Downstate
       Medical Center
       Brooklyn, New York   11203

50.   State University of New York Upstate
       Medical Center
       Syracuse, New York   13210

51.   Temple University Health Sciences Center
       School of Medicine
       Philadelphia, Pennsylvania   19140

52.   Texas Tech University School of Medicine
       Lubbock, Texas   79409

53.   Tufts University School of Medicine
       New Orleans, Louisiana   70112

55.   Uniformed Services University of the Health Services
       School of Medicine
       Bethesda, Maryland   20014

56.   University of Alabama School of Medicine
       Birmingham, Alabama   35233

57.   University of Alberta Faculty of Medicine
       Edmonton, Alberta T6G 2E1, Canada

58.   University of Arizona College of Medicine
       Tucson, Arizona 85724

59.   University of Arkansas for Medical Sciences
       Little Rock, Arkansas   72201

60.   University of California at Davis
       School of Medicine
       Davis, California   95616

61.   University of California at Irvine
       California College of Medicine
       Irvine, California   92664

62.   University of California at Los Angeles
       School of Medicine
       Los Angeles, California   90024

63.   University of San Diego
       School of Medicine
       La Jolia, California   92093

64.   University of California at San Francisco

San Francisco, California 94143
65. University of California at San Francisco
School of Medicine
San Francisco, California 94143
66. University of Chicago
Pritzker School of Medicine
Chicago, Illinois 60637
67. University of Cincinnati College of Medicine
Cincinnati, Ohio 45267
68. University of Colorado Health Sciences Center
Graduate School, Department of Medicine
Denver, Colorado 80262
69. University of Connecticut Health Center
College of Medicine
Farmington, Connecticut 06032
70. University of Florida College of Medicine
Gainesville, Florida 32601
71. University of Hawaii School of Medicine
Honolulu, Hawaii 96816
72. University of Health Sciences
Chicago Medical School
Chicago, Illinois 60612
73. University of Illinois Medical Center
Chicago, Illinois 60612
74. University of Iowa College of Medicine Center
Iowa City, Iowa 52240
75. University of Kansas Medical Center
College of Health Sciences
School of Medicine
Kansas City, Kansas 66103
76. University of Kentucky College of Medicine
Lexington, Kentucky 40506
77. University of Louisville Health Science Center
School of Medicine
Louisville, Kentucky 40208
78. University of Maryland School of Medicine
Baltimore, Maryland 21201
79. University of Massachusetts Medical School
Worcester, Massachusetts 01605
80. University of Miami, School of Medicine
Miami, Florida 33152

81.   University of Michigan Medical School
       Ann Arbor, Michigan
82.   University of Minnesota
       School of Medicine
       Duluth, Minnesota 55812
83.   University of Minnesota
       Mayo Graduate School of Medicine
       Rochester, Minnesota 53901
84.   University of Minnesota Medical School
       Minneapolis, Minnesota 55455
85.   University of Mississippi Medical Center
       Jackson, Mississippi 39216
86.   University of Missouri-Columbia
       School of Medicine
       Columbia, Missouri 65201
87.   University of Missouri-Kansas City
       School of Medicine
       Kansas City, Missouri 54110
88.   University of Montreal Faculty of Medicine
       Montreal, Quebec H35 1J4, Canada
89.   University of Nebraska Medical Center
       Omaha, Nebraska 68105
90.   University of New Mexico School of Medicine
       Albuquerque, New Mexico 27514
91.   University of North Carolina School of Medicine
       Chapel Hill, North Carolina 27514
92.   University of North Dakota School of Medicine
       Grand Forks, North Dakota 58201
93.   University of Oklahoma Health Sciences Center
       Oklahoma City, Oklahoma 73190
94.   University of Oregon Health Sciences Center
       Portland, Oregon 97201
95.   University of Pennsylvania School of Medicine
       Philadelphia, Pennsylvania 15261
96.   University of Pittsburgh School of Medicine
       Pittsburgh, Pennsylvania 15261
97.   University of Puerto Rico School of Medicine
       San Juan, Puerto Rico 00905
98.   University of Rochester
       School of Medicine and Dentistry
       Department of Medicine

Rochester, New York   14642

99.   University of South Alabama College of Medicine
Mobile, Alabama   36688

100.   University of South Carolina School of Medicine
Columbia, South Carolina   29208

101.   University of South Dakota School of Medicine
Vermillion, South Dakota   57069

102.   University of Southern California School of Medicine
Los Angeles, California   90033

103.   University of South Florida College of Medicine
Tampa, Florida   33620

104.   University of Tennessee Center for the Health Sciences
Memphis, Tennessee   38163

105.   University of Texas Medical Branch at Galveston
Galveston, Texas   77550

106.   University of Texas Medical School
Houston, Texas   77025

107.   University of Texas Medical School
San Antonio, Texas   78284

108.   University of Texas Southwestern Medical School
Dallas, Texas   75235

109.   University of Utah College of Medicine
Salt Lake City, Utah   84132

110.   University of Vermont College of Medicine
Burlington, Vermont   05401

111.   University of Virginia School of Medicine
Charlottesville, Virginia   22901

112.   University of Washington School of Medicine
Seattle, Washington   98105

113.   University of Western Ontario Faculty of Medicine
London, Ontario N6A 3K7, Canada

114.   University of Wisconsin Medical School
Madison, Wisconsin   53706

115.   Vanderbilt University School of Medicine
Nashville, Tennessee   37203

116.   Virginia Commonwealth University
Medical College of Virginia
Richmond, Virginia   23298

117.   Wake Forest University
Bowman Gray School of Medicine
Winston-Salem, North Carolina   27103

118.   Washington University School of Medicine
        St. Louis, Missouri   63110
119.   Wayne State University School of Medicine
        Detroit, Michigan   48201
120.   West Virginia University School of Medicine
        Morgantown, West Virginia   26506
121.   Wright State University School of Medicine
        North Dayton, Ohio   45431
122.   Yale University School of Medicine
        New Haven, Connecticut   06520
123.   Yeshiva University
        Albert Einstein College of Medicine
        Bronx, New York   10461

Archives

1. Department of Archives and History
    624 Washington Avenue
    Montgomery, Alabama   36130
2. Division of General Service and Supply
    Department of Administration
    Pouch C
    Juneau, Alaska   99811
3. Department of Libraries, Archives and Public Records
    State Capitol, 3rd Floor
    Phoenix, Arizona   85007
4. History Commission
    Department of Parks and Tourism
    One Capitol Mall
    Little Rock, Arkansas   72201
5. State Archives
    Office of the Secretary of State
    1230 J Street
    Sacramento, California   95814
6. Archives and Public Records
    Department of Administration
    Centennial Building, 1B
    Denver, Colorado   80203
7. State Library
    231 Capitol Avenue
    Hartford, Connecticut   06115
8. Department of State
    Hall of Records
    Dover, Delaware   19901
9. Division of Archives, History and Records Management
    Department of State
    R. A. Gray Building
    Tallahassee, Florida   32301
10. Archives and Records
    Office of the Secretary of State
    330 Capitol Avenue SE
    Atlanta, Georgia   30334
11. Department of Accounting and General Services
    Iolani Palace Grounds
    Honolulu, Hawaii   96813

12.   State Archives
        State Board of Education
        325 West State Street
        Boise, Idaho 83720
13.   Division of Archives and Records
        Office of the Secretary of State
        Archives Building
        Springfield, Illinois 62706
14.   Commission of Public Records
        State Library
        140 North Senate Avenue
        Indianapolis, Indiana 46204
15.   Division of History Museum and Archives
        Historical Department
        Historical Building
        Des Moines, Iowa 50319
16.   State Historical Society
        210 West Tenth Street
        Topeka, Kansas 66612
17.   Division of Archives and Records
        Department of Library and Archives
        851 East Main Street
        Frankfort, Kentucky 40601
18.   Division of Archives
        Department of State
        PO Box 44125
        Baton Rouge, Louisiana 70804
19.   State Archives
        Office of the Secretary of State
        State House, Station 84
        Augusta, Maine 04333
20.   Hall of Records
        College Avenue & St. John's Street
        PO Box 828
        Annapolis, Maryland 21404
21.   Office of Secretary of Commonwealth
        State House, Room 55
        Boston, Massachusetts 02133
22.   Division of Michigan History
        208 North Capitol
        Lansing, Michigan 48918

23. Division of Archives and Manuscripts
Historical Society
1500 Mississippi Street
St. Paul, Minnesota 55101
24. Department of Archives and History
PO Box 571
Jackson, Mississippi 39201
25. Records Management and Archives Service
Office of Secretary of State
1001 Industrial Drive
Jefferson City, Missouri 65102
26. Records Management and Archives Service
Office of the Secretary of State
PO Box 778
Jefferson City, Missouri 65102
27. Historical Society
Board of Education
225 North Roberts
Helena, Montana 59620
28. Historical Society
1500 R Street
Lincoln, Nebraska 68508
29. State Library
401 North Carson Street
Carson City, Nevada 89710
30. Division of Records Management and Archives
Department of State
71 South Fruit Street
Concord, New Hampshire 03301
31. State Library, Archives and History
Department of Education
185 West State Street, CN-5202
Trenton, New Jersey 08625
32. State Records and Archive Center
404 Montezuma Avenue
Santa Fe, New Mexico 87503
33. Cultural Education Center
Empire State Plaza, Room 10A46
Albany, New York 12230
34. Division of Archives and History
Department of Cultural Resources

109 East Jones Street
Raleigh, North Carolina   27611
35.   Historical Society
Heritage Center Building, Capital Grounds
Bismarck, North Dakota   59505
36.   Division of Archives and Manuscripts
Historical Society
1982 Velma Avenue
Columbus, Ohio   43211
37.   Department of Libraries
200 NE 18th
Oklahoma City, Oklahoma   73105
38.   Division of Archives
Office of the Secretary of State
1005 Broadway NE
Salem, Oregon   97310
39.   Bureau of Archives and History
Historical and Museum Commission
A-26 Archives Building
Harrisburg, Pennsylvania   17120
40.   Division of Archives
Office of the Secretary of State
43 State House
Providence, Rhode Island   02903
41.   Department of Archives and History
1430 Senate Street
PO Box 11669
Columbia, South Carolina   29211
42.   Division of Cultural Preservation
Education and Cultural Affairs
Kneip Building
Pierre, South Dakota   57501
43.   Division of Library and Archives
Department of Education
403 Seventh Avenue North
Nashville, Tennessee   37219
44.   Division of Archives
State Library and Archives Commission
PO Box 12927, Capitol Station
Austin, Texas   78711
45.   State Capitol, B-4

Salt Lake City, Utah   84114
46.   Division of Public Records
      Agency of Administration
      State Administration Building
      Montpelier, Vermont   05602
47.   State Library
      11th & Capitol Station
      Richmond, Virginia   23219
48.   Archives and Records Management
      Office of the Secretary of State
      12th & Washington Street
      Olympia, Washington   98504
49.   Division of Archives and History
      Department of Culture and History
      Science and Culture Center
      Charleston, West Virginia   25305
50.   Division of Archives
      Historical Society
      816 State Street
      Madison, Wisconsin   53706
51.   Department of Archives, Museums, and History
      Barrett Building
      Cheyenne, Wyoming   82001
52.   Ponce de Leon 500
      Puerta de Tierra
      San Juan, Puerto Rico   00905

Health Libraries

1.   Association of American Medical Colleges
        Archives Department
        One Dupont Circle NW
        Washington, D.C.
2.   Booth Memorial Medical Center
        Medical Library
        Main Street at South Memorial Avenue
        Flushing, New York
3.   Boston City Hospital
        Medical Library
        818 Harrison Avenue
        Boston, Massachusetts
4.   Boston City Hospital-Nursing
        Morse Slanger
        35 Northampton Street
        Boston, Massachusetts
5.   Boston University Library
        Boston University
        Department of Special Collection
        771 Common Wealth Avenue
        Boston, Massachusetts
6.   California State
        Department of Health Sciences Library
        2151 Berkeley Way
        Berkeley, California
7.   Catholic Medical Center of Brooklyn and Queens, Inc.
        Saint Mary's Hospital-Medical Library
        1298 Saint Mark's Avenue
        Brooklyn, New York
8.   Catholic University of America
        Health Science Library
        Washington, D. C.
9.   Chicago Institute for Psychoanalysis
        180 North Michigan
        Chicago, Illinois
10.   Children's Memorial Hospital Library
        2300 Children's Plaza
        Chicago, Illinois
11.   Cleveland Health Sciences Library

2119 Abington Road
Cleveland, Ohio
12. Cook County Hospital-Frederick Tice Hospital
720 South Wolcott Street
Chicago, Illinois
13. Deaconess Hospital-Drusch Professional Library
6150 Oakland Avenue
St. Louis, Missouri
14. Denver Medical Society Library
1601 East 19th Avenue
Denver, Colorado
15. Maine Medical Center-Health Sciences Library
22 Bramhall Street
Portland, Maine
16. Eagleville Hospital and Rehabilitation Center
Henry S. Loucheem Medical Library
Box 45
Eagleville, Pennsylvania
17. Emory University-School of Dentistry
Sheppard W. Foster Library
1462 Clifton Road NE
Atlanta, Georgia
18. Framingham Union Hospital
Cesare George Tedeschi Library
Evergreen Street
Framingham, Massachusetts
19. Gateways Hospital and Community Mental Health Center
Professional Library
1891 Effie Street
Los Angeles, California
20. Georgia State Department of Human Resources
Georgia Mental Health Institute
Addison M. DuVal Library
1256 Briarcliff Road NE
Atlanta, Georgia
21. Graduate Hospital Library
One Graduate Plaza
Philadelphia, Pennsylvania
22. Harkness Eye Institute
John M. Wheeler Library
635 West 165th Street

New York, New York
23.   Harlem Hospital Center-Library
       506 Lenox Avenue
       New York, New York
24.   Hartford Hospital-Health Sciences Libraries
       80 Seymour Street
       Hartford, Connecticut
25.   Institute for Cancer Research Library
       7701 Burholme Avenue, Fox Chase
       Philadelphia, Pennsylvania
26.   Jefferson University Cardeza Foundation
       Tocantings Memorial Library
       1015 Walnut Street
       Philadelphia, Pennsylvania
27.   Lindemann (Erich) Mental Health Center Library
       Government Center
       Boston, Massachusetts
28.   Los Angeles County Medical Association Library
       634 South West Lake Avenue
       Los Angeles, California
29.   Medical and Chirurgical Facility of the State of Maryland Library
       1211 Cathedral Street
       Baltimore, Maryland
30.   Memorial Sloan-Kettering Cancer Center
       Lee Coombe Memorial Library
       1275 York Avenue
       New York, New York
31.   Mid-Maine Medical Center
       Clara Hodgkins Memorial Health Science Laboratory
       Waterville, Main
32.   New York City-Municipal Reference and Research Center
       Hoven Emerson Public Health Library
       125 Worth Street, Room 223
       New York, New York
33.   Newark Beth Israel Medical Center Drive
       Victor Paesonnet Memorial Library
       201 Lyons Avenue
       Newark, New Jersey
34.   Norton-Children's Hospital Medical Library
       Box 35070
       Louisville, Kentucky

35.   Philadelphia State Hospital
      Staff Library Research-Education Building
      14000 Roosevelt Boulevard
      Philadelphia, Pennsylvania
36.   Rhode Island Hospital-Peterson Memorial Library
      Providence, Rhode Island
37.   Saint Joseph Hospital Library
      213 East Alta Vista
      Ottumwa, Iowa
38.   St. Louis Metropolitan Medical Society
      St. Louis Society for Medical & Scientific
      Education Library
      3839 Lindell Boulevard
      St. Louis, Missouri
39.   Saint Vincent Charity Hospital Library
      2351 East 22nd Street
      Cleveland, Ohio
40.   San Francisco-Psychoanalytic Institute-Library
      2420 Sutter Street
      San Francisco, California
41.   Slavonic Benevolent Order of the State of Texas
      Library, Archives, Museum
      520 North Main Street
      Temple, Texas
42.   South Hills Health System
      Behan Health Science Library
      Coal Valley Road, Box 18119
      Pittsburgh, Pennsylvania
43.   Touro Infirmary-Hospital Library
      1401 Toucher Street, Room 102
      M. Building
      New Orleans, Louisiana
44.   Ukrainian Medical Association of North America
      Medical Archives and Library
      2453 West Chicago Avenue
      Chicago, Illinois
45.   U. S. Public Health Service Hospital
      Gallop Indian Medical Center-Medical Library
      East Nizhilni Boulevard, Box 1337
      Gallup, New Mexico
46.   U. S. Public Health Service Hospital

Phoenix Indiana Medical Center Library
4212 North 16th Street
Phoenix, Arizona
47.   White Memorial Medical Center
1720 Brooklyn Avenue
Los Angeles, California
48.   Wilcox Memorial Hospital and Health Center
Medical Library
3420 Kuhio Hox
Lihue, Hawaii

Ethnic Libraries

1. African Bibliographic Center
    Staff Resource Library
    1346 Connecticut Avenue NW, Room 901
    Washington, DC   20036
2. Afro-American Cultural and Historical Society Museum
    1839 East 81st Street
    Cleveland, Ohio   44103
3. American Indian Historical Society-Library
    1451 Masonic Avenue
    San Francisco, California   94117
4. Appalachian Cultural Resources Center and Library
    Bule Ridge Parkway
    Box 9098, Oteen
    Ashville, North Carolina   28805
5. Arizona State University
    Arizona Collection-Chicano Studies Library Project
    Hayden Library
    Tempe, Arizona   85281
6. Association of the Study of Afro-American Life and History Library
    1401 14th Street NW
    Washington, DC   20005
7. Atlanta University
    Trevor Arnett Library
    273 Chestnut Street SW
    Atlanta, Georgia   30314
8. Bennett College
    Thomas F. Holgate Library
    Greensboro, North Carolina   27420
9. California Institute of Asian Studies-Library
    3494 21st Street
    San Francisco, California   94110
10. Cherokee National Historical Society, Inc.
    Library and Archives
    Box 515
    TSA-LA-G1
    Tahlequah, Oklahoma   74464
11. Cherokee Regional Library
    Georgia History and Genealogical Room
    305 South Duke Street

LaFayette, Georgia 30728
12. Chicago Public Library Cultural Center
Vivian G. Harsh Collection of Afro-American History and Literature
9525 South Haister Street
Chicago, Illinois 60628
13. Chinese Cultural Center-Library
159 Lexington Avenue
New York, New York 10016
14. Cornell University
Africana Studies and Research Center Library
310 Triphammer Road
Ithaca, New York 14853
15. District of Columbia Public Library
Black Studies Division
Martin Luther King Memorial Library
901 G Street NW
Washington, DC 20001
16. Du Sable Museum of African American History-Library
740 East 56th P.
Chicago, Illinois 60637
17. Huntington Free Library
9 Westchester Square
Bronx, New York 10461
18. Johnson Publishing Company, Inc.-Library
820 South Michigan Avenue
Chicago, Illinois 60605
19. Kossuth Fundation-Hungarian Research Library
Butler University
Indianapolis, Indiana 46208
20. Langston University
Melvine E. Tolson Black Heritage Center
Second Floor, Page Hall Annex
Langston, Oklahoma 73050
21. Library of Congress-American Folklife Center
Thomas Jefferson Building, G1040
Washington, DC 20540
22. Library of Congress-Asian Division
John Adams Building, Room 1024
Washington, DC 20540
23. Library of Congress- Hispanic Division
Thomas Jefferson Building, Room 239E

Washington, DC   20540
24.   Lincoln University
       Lanston Hughes Memorial Library-Special Collection
       Lincoln University, Pennsylvania   19352
25.   Lloyd (Alice) College
       Appalachian Oral History Project
       Pippa Passes, Kentucky   41844
26.   Michigan State University-International Library
       W310-316 University Library
       East Lansing, Michigan   48824
27.   Museum of Indian Heritage-Library
       Eagle Creek Park
       6040 DeLong Road
       Indianapolis, Indiana   46254
28.   National Association Pro Spanish Speaking Elderly
       Library
       3875 Wilshire Boulevard, Suite 401
       Los Angeles, California   90010
29.   National Indian Education Association-Library
       Ivy Tower Building, Second Floor
       1115 Second Avenue South
       Minneapolis, Minnesota   55403
30.   Navajo Nation Library
       Box K
       Window Rock, Arizona   86515
31.   Oakland Public Library-Asian Community Library
       125 14th Street
       Oakland, California   94612
32.   Oakland Public Library-Latin American Library
       1900 Fruitvale Avenue, Suite 1-A
       Oakland, California   94601
33.   Ohio State University-Black Studies Library
       1858 Nei Avenue
       Columbus, Ohio   43210
34.   Ohio State University-East Asian Collection
       1858 Nei Avenue
       Columbus, Ohio   43210
35.   Oklahoma Historical Society
       Chickasaw Council House Library
       Court House Square
       Tishomingo, Oklahoma   73460

36.   Ponca City Cultural Center Museum-Library
       1000 East Grand Street
       Ponca City, Oklahoma 74601
37.   Queens Borough Public Library
       Langston Hughes Library and Cultural Center
       102-09 Northern Boulevard
       Corona, New York 11368
38.   Seattle Public Library-Douglas-Truth Branch Library
       23rd Avenue & East Yesier Way
       Seattle, Washington 98122
39.   Slavonic Benevolent Order of the State of Texas
       Library, Archives, Museum
       520 North Main Street
       Temple, Texas 76501
40.   Swedish Pioneer Archives
       5125 North Spaulding Avenue
       Chicago, Illinois 60625
41.   Tuskegee Institute
       Hollis Burke Frissell Library-Archives
       Tuskegee Institute, Alabama 36088
42.   U. S. Public Health Service Hospital
       Gallup Indian Medical Center-Medical Library
       East Nizhoni Boulevard, Box 1337
       Gallup, New Mexico 84301
43.   University Boricua
       Puerto Rican Research and Resources Center, Inc.
       Reference Library
       1766 Church Street
       Washington, DC 20036
44.   University of Alaska-Alaska Native Language Center
       Research Library
       302 Chapman Building
       Fairbanks, Alaska 99701
45.   University of Alaska
       Alaska and the Polar Regions Collection
       Elmer E. Rasmuston Library
       Fairbanks, Alaska 99701
46.   University of California-Berkeley
       Asian American Studies Library
       3407 Dwinelle Hall
       Berkeley, California 94720

47. University of California-Berkeley
     Native American Studies Library
     343 Dwinelle Hall
     Berkeley, California   94720
48. University of Massachusetts
     Amherst University Archives
     University Library
     Amherst, Massachusetts   01002
49. University of Puerto Rico-Puerto Rican Collection
     Box C. U. P. R. Station
     Ric Piedras, Puerto Rico   00931
50. University of Washington-Special Collections Division
     Pacific Northwest Collection
     Suzzallo Library, FM-25
     Seattle, Washington   98195
51. Yale University-American Oriental Society Library
     Sterling Memorial Library, Room 329
     New Haven, Connecticut   06520
52. Canada-Indian and Northern Affairs
     Canada-Departmental Library
     Terrasses De La Chaudiere
     Ottawa Ontario, K1A DH4 Canada

Minority College Libraries

1.   Alabama Agricultural and Mechanical University
        Normal, Alabama   35762
2.   Alabama State University
        Montgomery, Alabama   36195
3.   Albany State College
        Albany, Georgia   31705
4.   Alcorn State University
        Lorman, Mississippi   39096
5.   Allen University
        Columbia, South Carolina   29204
6.   Arkansas Baptist College
        Little Rock, Arkansas   72501
7.   Atlanta University
        Atlanta, Georgia   30314
8.   Barker-Scolta College
        Concord, North Carolina   28025
9.   Benedict College
        Columbia, South Carolina   29204
10.   Bethune-Cookman College
        Daytona Beach, Florida   32015
11.   Bishop College
        Dallas, Texas   75241
12.   Bluefield State College
        Bluefield, West Virginia   24701
13.   Bowie State College
        Bowie, Maryland   20715
14.   Central State University
        Wilberforce, Ohio   45384
15.   Cheyney State College
        Cheyney, Pennsylvania   19319
16.   Claflin University
        Orangeburg, South Carolina   29115
17.   Clark College
        Atlanta, Georgia   30314
18.   Coahoma Junior College
        Clarksdale, Mississippi   38614
19.   College of the Virgin Islands-St. Thomas
        St. Thomas, Virgin Islands   00801
20.   Coppin State College

Baltimore, Maryland   21216
21.   Daniel Payne College
      Birmingham, Alabama   35212
22.   Delaware State College
      Dover, Delaware   19901
23.   Dillard University
      New Orleans, Louisiana   70122
24.   D. C. Teachers College
      Washington, DC   20003
25.   Edward Walters College
      Jacksonville, Florida   32209
26.   Elizabeth State College
      Elizabeth City, North Carolina   27909
27.   Fayetteville State University
      Fayetteville, North Carolina   28301
28.   Federal City College
      Washington, DC   20005
29.   Fisk University
      Nashville, Tennessee   37203
30.   Florida A & M University
      Tallahassee, Florida   32307
31.   Florida Memorial College
      Miami, Florida   33054
32.   Fort Valley State College
      Fort Valley, Georgia   31030
33.   Grambling College
      Grambling, Louisiana   71245
34.   Hampton Institute
      Hampton, Virginia   23668
35.   Huston-Fillotson College
      Austin, Texas   78702
36.   Jackson State College
      Jackson, Mississippi   39217
37.   Jarvis Christian College
      Hawkins, Texas   75765
38.   Johnson C. Smith College
      Charlotte, North Carolina   28216
39.   Kentucky State College
      Frankfort, Kentucky   40601
40.   Kitrell College
      Kitrell, North Carolina   27544

41. Knoxville College
     Knoxville, Tennessee 37921
42. Lane College
     Jackson, Tennessee 28301
43. Langston University
     Langston, Oklahoma 73050
44. Lemoyne-Owen College
     Memphis, Tennessee 38126
45. Lincoln University
     Jefferson City, Missouri 65101
46. Lincoln University
     Lincoln University, Pennsylvania 19352
47. Lelvingstone College
     Salisbury, North Carolina 28144
48. Lomax-Nannon Junior College
     Greenville, Alabama 36037
49. Mary Holmes College
     West Point, Mississippi 39773
50. Miles College
     Birmingham, Alabama 35208
51. Mississippi Valley State College
     Itta Bena, Mississippi 38941
52. Mississippi Industrial College
     Holly Springs, Mississippi 38635
53. Mobile State Junior College
     Mobile, Alabama 36613
54. Morehouse College
     Atlanta, Georgia 30314
55. Morgan State University
     Baltimore, Maryland 21239
56. Morris Brown College
     Atlanta, Georgia 30314
57. Morris College
     Sumter, South Carolina 29150
58. Morristown College
     Morristown, Tennessee 37814
59. Natchez Junior College
     Natchez, Mississippi 39120
60. Norfolk State College
     Norfolk, Virginia 23504
61. North Carolina Central University

Durham, North Carolina 27707
62. Oakwood College
Huntsville, Alabama 35806
63. Paine College
Augusta, Georgia 30910
64. Paul Quinn College
Waco, Texas 76704
65. Philander Smith College
Little Rock, Arkansas 72203
66. Prairie View A & M University
Prairie View, Texas 77445
67. Rust College
Holly Springs, Mississippi 38635
68. St. Augustine's College
Raleigh, North Carolina 27611
69. Savannah State College
Savannah, Georgia 31404
70. Selma University
Selma, Alabama 36701
71. Shaw University
Raleigh, North Carolina 27611
72. Shorter College
North Little Rock, Alabama 72114
73. Simmon's University
Louisville, Kentucky 40210
74. S. C. State College
Orangeburg, South Carolina 29117
75. Southern University A & M College
Baton Rouge, Louisiana 70813
76. Southwestern Christian College
Terrell, Texas 75160
77. Spelman College
Atlanta, Georgia 30314
78. Stillman College
Tuscaloosa, Alabama 35401
79. Talladega College
Talladega, Alabama 35160
80. Tennessee State University
Nashville, Tennessee 37203
81. Texas College
Tyler, Texas 75701

82.   Texas Southeast University
       Houston, Texas   77004
83.   Theodore Alfred Lawson State Junior College
       Birmingham, Alabama   35228
84.   Tougaloo College
       Tougaloo, Mississippi   35228
85.   Tuskegee Institute
       Tuskegee Institute, Alabama   36088
86.   University of Arkansas at Pine Bluff
       Pine Bluff, Arkansas   71601
87.   University of D. C.
       Washington, DC
88.   University of Maryland Eastern Shore
       Princess Anne, Maryland   21853
89.   Utica Junior College
       Utica, Mississippi   39175
90.   Virginia State College
       Petersburg, Virginia   23803
91.   Virginia Union University
       Richmond, Virginia   23220
92.   Voorhees College
       Denmark, South Carolina   29042
93.   West Virginia State College
       Institute, West Virginia   25112
94.   Wilberforce University
       Wilberforce, Ohio   45384
95.   Wiley College
       Marshall, Texas   75670
96.   Winston-Salem State University
       Winston-Salem, North Carolina   27162
97.   Xavier University of Louisiana
       New Orleans, Louisiana   70125
98.   Alabama Lutheran Academy & College
       Selma, Alabama   36701
99.   Bronx Community College
       New York, New York
100.   Chicago State University
       Chicago, Illinois   60628
101.   Chicago Theological Seminary
       Chicago, Illinois
102.   Clinton Junior College

Rock Hill, South Carolina 29730
103. Detroit Institute of Technology
      Detroit, Michigan 48201
104. Compton College
      Los Angeles, California 90221
105. Kennedy-King College
      Chicago, Illinois 60621
106. Los Angeles Southwest College
      Los Angeles, California 90047
107. Malcom-King; Harlem College Extension
      103 East 125th Street
      New York, New York 10035
108. Malcom X College
      Chicago, Illinois 60612
109. Manhattanville College
      Pusckase, New York
110. Mary Allan Junior College
      Crockette, Texas 75835
111. Martin Technical Institute
      Williamston, North Carolina 27892
112. Medgar Evers Community College
      New York City, New York
113. North Carolina A & T State University
      Greensboro, North Carolina 27411
114. Olive-Harvey College
      Chicago, Illinois 60628
115. Saints College
      Lexington, Mississippi 39095
116. St. Paul's College
      Lawrenceville, Virginia 23868
117. S. D. Bishop State Junior College
      Mobile, Alabama 36603
118. Virginia College
      Lynchburg, Virginia 24501
119. Washington Technical Institute
      Washington, DC 20008
120. Wayne County Community College
      Detroit, Michigan 48201
121. Westfield State College
      Westfield, Maryland

Hospitals

1.   Provident Hospital
        51st Street
        Chicago, Illinois   60615
2.   Norfolk Community Hospital
        2539 Corprew Avenue
        Norfolk, Virginia   23504
3.   Whittaker Memorial Hospital
        Box 538
        Newport News, Virginia   23607
4.   Lincoln Hospital
        234 East 149th Street
        Bronx, New York   10451
5.   Mercy Hospital
        Landondown Avenue and Baily Road
        Darby, Pennsylvania   19023
6.   Flint-Goodridge Hospital
        2425 Louisiana Avenue
        New Orleans, Louisiana   70115

Medical Associations

1. Medical-Chirurgical Society of the District of Columbia
    1310 Pennsylvania Avenue NW
    Washington, DC
2. National Medical Association
    1301 Pennsylvania Avenue
    Washington, DC   20037
3. National Dental Association
    PO Box 197
    Charlottesville, Virginia   22902
4. American Nursing Association
    2420 Pershing Road
    Kansas City, Missouri   64108
5. U. S. Information Agency
    National Archives
    Washington, DC   20408
6. American Medical Association
    535 North Dearborn Street
    Chicago, Illinois   60610
7. American Black Nurses Association
    PO Box 18358
    Boston, Massachusetts   02118

Public Libraries (25 Largest U. S. Cities)

1.   Phoenix Public Library
      12 East McDowell Road
      Phoenix, Arizona   80054
2.   Los Angeles Public Library
      630 West Fifth Street
      Los Angeles, California   90017
3.   San Diego Public Library
      820 E Street
      San Diego, California   92101
4.   San Francisco Public Library
      Civic Center
      San Francisco, California   94102
5.   San Jose Public Library
      180 West San Carlos Street
      San Jose, California   95113
6.   Denver Public Library
      1357 Broadway
      Denver, Colorado   80203
7.   District of Columbia Public Library
      901 G Street
      Washington, DC   20001
8.   Jacksonville Public Library
      122 North Ocean Street
      Jacksonville, Florida   32202
9.   Hawaii State Library System
      478 South King Street
      Honolulu, Hawaii   96813
10.   Chicago Public Library
      78 East Washington Street
      Chicago, Illinois   60602
11.   Indianapolis-Marion County Public Library
      40 E Street
      Indianapolis, Indiana   46204
12.   New Orleans Public Library
      219 Loyola Avenue
      New Orleans, Louisiana   70140
13.   Enoch Pratt Free Library
      400 Cathedral Street
      Baltimore, Maryland   21201

14.   Boston Public Library
      Copley Square
      Boston, Massachusetts 02116
15.   Detroit Pubilc Library
      5201 Woodward Avenue
      Detroit, Michigan 48202
16.   New York City Public Library
      Fifth Avenue at 42nd Street
      New York, New York 10018
17.   Cleveland Public Library
      325 Superior Avenue
      Cleveland, Ohio 44114
18.   Columbus Public Library
      96 South Grant Avenue
      Columbus, Ohio 43215
19.   Philadelphia Free Library
      Logan Square
      Philadelphia, Pennsylvania 19103
20.   Memphis Public Library
      258 South McLean Boulevard
      Memphis, Tennessee 38104
21.   Dallas Public Library
      1954 Commerce Street
      Dallas, Texas 75201
22.   Houston Public Library
      Civic Center
      500 McKinney Avenue
      Houston, Texas 77002
23.   San Antonio Public Library
      203 South St. Mary's
      San Antonio, Texas 78205
24.   Seattle Public Library
      1000 Fourth Avenue
      Seattle, Washington 98104
25.   Milwaukee Public Library
      814 West Wisconsin Avenue
      Milwaukee, Wisconsin 53133

Government Agencies

1.   Health Services Administration
        5600 Fishers Lane
        Rockville, Maryland   20857
2.   National Institutes of Health
        9000 Rockville Pike
        Bethesda, Maryland   20205
3.   National Cancer Institute
        9000 Rockville Pike
        Bethesda, Maryland   20205
4.   Health Care Financing Administration
        Department of Health and Human Service
        330 C Street SW
        Washington, DC   20201
5.   National Heart, Lung, and Blood Institute
        9000 Rockville Pike
        Bethesda, Maryland   20205
6.   National Institute of Allergy and Infectious Disease
        9000 Rockville Pike
        Bethesda, Maryland   20205
7.   National Institute of Arthritis, Diabetes and Kidney Disease
        9000 Rockville Pike
        Bethesda, Maryland   20205
8.   Department of Agriculture
        14th Street and Independence Avenue SW
        Washington, DC   20205
9.   National Institute on Aging
        9000 Rockville Pike
        Bethesda, Maryland   20205
10.   National Institute of Dental Research
        9000 Rockville Pike
        Bethesda, Maryland   20205
11.   National Institute of Environmental Health Sciences
        PO Box 12233
        Research Triangle Park, North Carolina   27709
12.   National Institute of General Medical Sciences
        Westwood Building, Room 9A12
        Bethesda, Maryland   20205
13.   National Institute of Neurological and Communicative Disorders and
        Stroke

9000 Rockville Pike
Bethesda, Maryland 20205

14. Office of Health and Human Services
Human Development Services
Humphrey Building
Washington, DC 20201

15. Government Printing Office
North Capitol and H Street NW
Washington, DC 20401

16. Center for Disease Control
1600 Clifton Road NE
Atlanta, Georgia 30333

17. Food and Drug Administration
5600 Fishers Lane
Rockville, Maryland 20857

18. Health Resources Administration
Center Building
3700 East-West Highway
Hyattsville, Maryland 20782

19. Library of Congress
10 First Street SW
Washington, DC 20540

20. Alcohol, Drug Abuse, and Mental Health Administration
5600 Fishers Lane
Rockville, Maryland 20857

21. National Center for Health Statistics
5600 Fishers Lane
Rockville, Maryland 20857

22. Health Services Administration
5600 Fishers Lane
Rockville, Maryland 20857

23. Health Care Financing Administration
330 C Street SW
Washington, DC 20201

24. Social Security Administration
6401 Security Boulevard
Baltimore, Maryland 21235

25. The Army Library
The Pentagon
Washington, DC 20310

26. The Navy Library

Department of the Navy
23rd and E Street NW
Washington, DC   20371

27.   The Library
        Uniformed Services University of Health Sciences
        4301 Jones Bridge Road
        Bethesda, Maryland   20014

28.   Air Force Magazine and Book Branch
        HQ USAF (SAF/OIPM)
        Washington, DC   20370

29.   Bureau of the Census
        Department of Commerce
        Washington, DC   20233

30.   National Resources Library
        Bureau of Indian Affairs
        Department of the Interior
        Washington, DC   20240

INDEX

About the Compiler

TYSON GIBBS is assistant professor of Anthropology at the University of North Texas.

ISBN 0-313-29740-1

90000>

EAN

9 780313 297403

HARDCOVER BAR CODE